The Cannabis
MIRACLE

107 Inspirational Stories of People Who Healed
Themselves Thanks to Cannabis

Published by
Inspired Publishing Ltd
27 Old Gloucester Street
London
WC1N 3AX

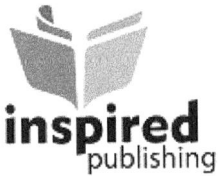
inspired publishing

Printed in the United Kingdom

ISBN : 978-1-78555-090-4

DISCLAIMER

The writer of this material believes that a natural and holistic approach to health and maintaining a balance within the human body are of extreme importance in experiencing energy, vitality, and vibrant health throughout life.

The author recognizes that within the scientific and medical fields there are widely divergent viewpoints and opinions. This material is written for the express purpose of sharing educational information and scientific research gathered from the studies and experiences of the author, healthcare professionals, scientists, nutritionists and informed health advocates.

None of the information contained in this book is intended to diagnose, prevent, treat, or cure any disease, nor is it intended to prescribe any of the techniques, materials or concepts presented as a form of treatment for any illness or medical condition.

Before beginning any practice relating to health, diet or exercise, it is highly recommended that you first obtain the consent and advice of a licensed health care professional.

The author assumes no responsibility for the choices you make after your review of the information contained herein and your consultation with a licensed healthcare professional.

None of the statements in this book have been evaluated by the Food & Drug Administration (FDA) or the American Medical Association (AMA).

DEDICATION

This book is dedicated to the tireless cannabis advocates who have made these remarkable stories of personal transformation and healing possible. May your stories inspire countless more to take back control of their lives and regain their health.

1

TABLE OF CONTENTS

Introduction 9

Chapter 1: Healing From Breast Cancer 13

Chapter 2: Healing From Colon Cancer 19

Chapter 3: Healing From Lung Cancer 35

Chapter 4: Healing From Skin Cancer, Melanomas, and Carcinomas 41

Chapter 5: Healing From Stomach and Bowel Cancer 53

Chapter 6: Healing From Kidney Cancer 63

Chapter 7: Healing From Bladder Cancer 67

Chapter 8: Healing From Liver Cancer 73

Chapter 9: Healing From Lymphoma 79

Chapter 10: Healing From Prostate Cancer 87

Chapter 11: Healing From Brain Cancer and Brain Tumours 91

Chapter 12: Healing From Leukaemia....................................103

Chapter 13: Other Types of Cancer.......................................111

Chapter 14: Epilepsy, Seizures and Cannabis 119

Chapter 15: Autism and Cannabis 139

Chapter 16: Cerebral Palsy and Cannabis 147

Chapter 17: Multiple Sclerosis and Cannabis 155

Chapter 18: Lyme Disease and Cannabis 159

Chapter 19: Inflammation, Chronic Pain, Fibromyalgia and Lupus 163

Chapter 20: Healing From Crohn's Disease, Colitis and Digestive Issues 179

Chapter 21: Healing From Glaucoma 189

Chapter 22: Amyotrophic Lateral Sclerosis and Cannabis 195

Chapter 23: Anxiety, Depression, PTSD, and Chronic Fatigue 199

Chapter 24: Alzheimer's and Parkinson's Disease....................211

Final Thoughts 221

News Headlines From Across The World

June 11, 2017 - Frances Bloomfield

Cannabis phytochemicals found to be effective in destroying leukemia cells

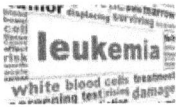

(Natural News) Researchers from St. George's, University of London have confirmed that cannabinoids are effective in destroying the cells of leukemia, a cancer of blood-forming organs. When used in conjunction with chemotherapy treatments, cannabinoids, the active chemicals in cannabis, results against the blood cancer cells improved ... [Read More...]

April 27, 2017 - Tracey Watson

CBD oil helps autistic boy speak again

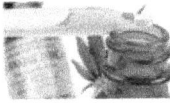

(Natural News) At first, when Kalel Santiago of Puerto Rico survived a rare form of cancer called neuroblastoma, his parents, Abiel and Gladys, were overjoyed that the two years of grueling surgery, radiation and chemotherapy treatments had worked, and their little boy was going to be okay. But while he was in the hospital, they started ... [Read More...]

4,210

DOCUMENTED: Cannabis extract successfully treats 14-year old girl with an "incurable" form of cancer

Tuesday, July 17, 2018 by: Vicki Batts
Tags: alternative medicine, cancer, cannabis, cannabis extract, cannabis oil, CBD, Chemotherapy, goodcancer, hemp, Herbs, leukemia, medical marijuana, natural cures, natural medicine

Cannabis oil with CBD saves child from epilepsy (while hospital doctors remain totally clueless)

Wednesday, June 08, 2016 by: Harold Shaw
Tags: cannabis oil, CBD, epilepsy

Cancer Survivor Says CBD Oil 'Saved Her Life' After Doctors Said She Had 6 Months To Live

Tuesday, September 12, 2017 by: News Editors
Tags: alternative medicine, cancer, cancer treatment, cannabis, CBD, CBD oil, hemp extracts

Cannabis oil (CBD) CURES 12-year-old girl of life-threatening seizures

Thursday, June 08, 2017 by: Amy Goodrich
Tags: cannabis, cannabis oil, CBD, CBD oil, Epilepsy, Febrile Infection-Related Epilepsy Syndrome, fires, Hemp Oil, herbal medicine, marijuana, natural cures, priority, seizures

CBD oil reduces chronic illness pain

Thursday, June 21, 2018 by: Vicki Batts
Tags: cannabidiol, cannabindoids, cannabis, CBD oil, chronic illnesses, chronic pain, goodhealth, goodmedicine, herbal medicine, natural medicine, natural remedies, pain relief, remedies, research

Cannabis reverses late-stage Alzheimer's

Tuesday, July 29, 2014 by: Paul Fassa
Tags: cannabis, Alzheimer''s, disease prevention

Cannabis found to reduce alcohol-induced liver disease, according to new study

Monday, January 29, 2018 by: Isabelle Z.
Tags: alcohol abuse, alcoholism, cannabis, cirrhosis, goodhealth, goodmedicine, goodscience, hemp, herbal medicine, inflammation, Liver cancer, liver damage, liver disease, liver health, medical marijuana, natural cures

Cannabis oil for chronic fatigue: A teenager says it cured his debilitating illness, has totally regained his quality of life after years of suffering

Thursday, January 04, 2018 by: Isabelle Z.
Tags: brain tumor, cannabis, cannabis oil, CBD, CBD oil, chronic fatigue, chronic fatigue syndrome, Epilepsy, goodhealth, goodmedicine, natural cures, natural medicine, natural remedies

Cannabis oil cures terminal cancer in 3-year-old after pharmaceutical drugs fail miserably

Thursday, October 29, 2015 by: Jennifer Lea Reynolds
Tags: cannabis oil, cancer treatment, Big Pharma

Cannabis beats "incurable" brain tumor after chemo fails

Thursday, September 14, 2017 by: Tracey Watson
Tags: brain tumor, cancer, cannabis, cannabis oil, CBD, Chemotherapy, incurable cancer, Lynn Cameron, medicinal herbs, natural cancer treatments, natural medicine, radiation

Cannabis oil is a highly efficient natural cancer cure

Wednesday, September 28, 2011 by: Raw Michelle
Tags: cannabis oil, cancer cure, health news

The State of Michigan declares cannabis legitimate medicine for treating arthritis, autism, chronic pain and more

Cannabis as a preventative: Studies show it helps guard against cancer, neurodegenerative disease, Alzheimer's, arthritis

Thursday, October 26, 2017 by: Zoey Sky
Tags: cannabis, Cures, hemp, medical marijuana, natural cures

Cannabis – Best Weapon Against the Brain Aging Process

Cannabis kicks Lyme disease to the curb

Wednesday, February 05, 2014 by: Paul Fassa
Tags: health news, Natural News, nutrition

Medical cannabis helps heal chronic disease

Thursday, June 19, 2014 by: Jonathan Landsman
Tags: medical cannabis, chronic disease, marijuana

Cannabis over chemo: Woman says the oil cured her aggressive breast cancer in 5 months

Wednesday, February 14, 2018 by: Isabelle Z.
Tags: breast cancer, cancer, cancer treatment, cannabis, cannabis oil, CBD, CBD oil, Chemotherapy, colon cancer, Cures, goodhealth, goodmedicine, leukemia, marijuana, medical marijuana, natural cures, natural medicine, natural remedies, remedies

Cannabis Beneficial for Multiple Sclerosis Patients, Study Finds

Saturday, February 06, 2010 by: Aaron Turpen
Tags: Cannabis, Multiple Sclerosis, health news

Cannabis more effective than prescriptions: Seventy-year-old grandmother threw out all her pills, says smoking cannabis manages her ailments

Wednesday, January 03, 2018 by: Russel Davis
Tags: cannabis, cannabis use, goodhealth, goodmedicine, herbal medicine, marijuana, medical marijuana, medicinal cannabis, natural medicine, natural remedies, smoking cannabis

Cannabis oil cures man's cancer after he was given 18 months to live

Tuesday, September 01, 2015 by: Jonathan Benson, staff writer
Tags: marijuana, cancer cure, cannabis

Cannabis dissolves cancerous tumor in young infant, deemed a 'miracle baby' by physician

Wednesday, September 24, 2014 by: Carolanne Wright
Tags: cannabis, cancerous tumors, miracle baby

INTRODUCTION

Patients from all over the world are reporting dramatic improvement from a multitude of conditions thanks to medicinal cannabis use.

Stomach cancer, Breast Cancer, Lung Cancer, Colon Cancer, Brain Tumours, Leukaemia, Lymphoma, Epilepsy, Seizures, Autism, Multiple Sclerosis, Lyme Disease, Inflammation, Chronic Pain, Arthritis, Ulcerative Colitis, Irritable Bowel Syndrome, Crohn's Disease, Glaucoma, Amyotrophic Lateral Sclerosis (ALS), Neuromuscular disorders, Parkinson's, and Alzheimer's—are just some of the ailments and illnesses that this miraculous plant has been shown to help heal.

In India, where cannabis has been used therapeutically for thousands of years, it was considered to be "the gift from the Gods," giving long life, renewing the mind, reducing fever, helping sleep, and curing dysentery.

As a result of sustained campaigning by health advocates in a number of countries, governments have—often reluctantly—started the process of legalizing cannabis for medicinal use, under strict guidelines. This has allowed companies to finally apply modern scientific research method-logies to exploring the healing properties of the 750 or more compounds contained within the cannabis plant.

My personal interest in the healing properties of this plant started when I came across the following article on the health-related website *NaturalNews.com.*

Researchers Have Known for Decades That Cannabis Kills Cancer Cells... Yet the Cover-Up Continues

"Since as early as 1974, researchers have known that THC, the active chemical in cannabis, shrinks or destroys tumours in rodents. Researchers at the Medical College of Virginia found that THC slowed the growth of three kinds of cancer in mice: lung and breast cancer, as well as virus-induced leukaemia. Without any mention in the mainstream media, the Drug Enforcement Administration (DEA) quickly shut down the study and destroyed its results.

Years later, researchers in Madrid confirmed these early results after successfully destroying incurable brain tumours in rats by injecting them with cannabinoids. They found that THC inhibits the growth of blood vessels that supply glucose to tumours, thereby halting tumour growth and prompting cancer cells to die-off.

To test for harmful biochemical or neurological effects, the Spanish researchers, led by Dr. Manuel Guzman of Complutense University, also administered large doses of THC to healthy rats. They found no adverse health effects. Again, no major U.S. newspapers ran this ground-breaking news.

There are still a lot of uncertainties about whether vaporizing or ingesting cannabis oil in combination with lifestyle and diet changes can be used as an alternative cancer treatment. But with many testimonials from those who have been helped, and several attempts to get cannabis oil allowed through the court system, the world might reach a conclusion soon.

As with many other promising natural treatments for cancer, research moves slowly, as the pharmaceutical cancer industry, backed up by governments, isn't too keen on shutting down its multi-billion-dollar chemotherapy business. They will do anything in their power to withhold the public from other, less damaging and cheaper cures.

While it is not recommended to feed your baby cannabis oil, a few years ago, **cannabinoid oil reduced the massive, centrally located and inoperable brain tumour of an 8-month-old within two months.** The child's father kept pushing Dr. William Courtney, who was quite sceptical about cannabis treatments, for non-traditional treatments based on marijuana. The baby was given cannabis oil via his pacifier, and was completely cured within eight months, as reported by *Organic and Healthy*.

After seeing the astonishing results with his own eyes, Dr. Courtney pointed out that the success of the cannabis approach means that children and adults no longer need to undergo the cruelties of surgery and long-term side effects that come from very high doses of chemotherapy or radiation."

Source: www.naturalnews.com/2017-01-30-researchers-have-known-for-decades-that-cannabis-kills-cancer-cells.html

Having written more than 40 books about alternative medicine since 2004 (mostly under a pen name), I was intrigued.

As I continued to research this topic, to my astonishment I came across hundreds of scientific studies confirming these findings. And yet the mainstream media were mostly silent about these breakthroughs.

What affected me the most while doing this research were the stories of people—and children, especially—who have healed themselves thanks to therapeutic properties of the cannabis plant, and the moving stories of their battle to regain their health.

In this book I have brought together a few of their stories (edited for conciseness), so that they may shine a light on a new path forwards for humanity, and bring you some inspiration, courage, and hope.

I believe this is the future of medicine.

I look forward to hearing your story, in due course, of your journey back to health – your very own "Cannabis Miracle."

CHAPTER 1

Healing From Breast Cancer

Can the Cannabis plant help women heal from Breast Cancer? In this chapter I share the stories of three women who definitely think so.

Case Study #1: Dee Mani Says Cannabis Oil Cured Her Aggressive Breast Cancer in 5 Months

"When Dee Mani, now 44, was diagnosed with breast cancer last March, her doctors suggested chemotherapy. She originally agreed to undergo one year of the treatment for her triple negative breast cancer – the deadliest type – but later had second thoughts. After seeing her sister suffer and die after undergoing chemotherapy for cancer, the mother of two set out to find an alternative.

She decided to take cannabis oil after researching natural cancer remedies online. She said she took one drop inside a capsule every night before going to bed because she didn't care for the taste or texture of it on its own. **Four months after her original diagnosis, her cancer had reduced significantly, and her doctors gave her the all-clear just five months after starting cannabis oil.**

She continues to take it to this day and says she plans to do so for the rest of her life as it has also helped her with problems like insomnia, allergy, and back pain. She has also changed her diet and taken up meditation."

Source: www.naturalnews.com/2018-02-14-cannabis-over-chemo-woman-says-the-oil-cured-her-aggressive-breast-cancer-in-5-months.html

Case Study #2: Stephanie LaRue Claims Cannabis Oil Saved Her Life

"Stephanie LaRue was diagnosed with breast cancer when she was only 30 years old. She underwent chemotherapy but was also looking for alternative cures.

She discovered and used Rick Simpson cannabis oil. After this, her cancer went into remission, and she has been a cancer survivor for over nine years now.

There is no scientific evidence that cannabis/hemp/Rick Simpson oil cures cancer in humans, but Stephanie herself believes that the oil saved her life."

Source: https://healthyhempoil.com/cannabis-oil-testimonial

Case Study #3: Breast Cancer Treated With Cannabis Extracts

"[I had] triple-Negative Breast Cancer Stage 4 with metastasis to the neck, left breast, lymph nodes, stomach and lungs. I was diagnosed in July 2014 and given two to three months to live. I was told radiation and surgery were impossible because of how far out the cancer had spread."

"I only wanted to do the [cannabis] oil and follow the organic and high alkaline diet, but the insurance would only cover my scans and blood work if I was being treated by the oncologist doing chemo. **I was mad because I was not given a choice, I felt forced to do chemo to have my progress covered.** I began Cannabis Oil two weeks before chemo was to start."

"My daughter did all the research on the chemo and per the FDA feedback and having gotten feedback from 3 other oncologists working mainly with Triple Negative patients, there was no way that any chemo would shrink or remove the tumours in my body. I began cannabis oil in early August 2014 and began chemo two weeks later. Chemo stopped at the end of December 2014."

"I was taking a daily multi vitamin. I had no symptoms of my stage 4 cancer. I had been working full time and feeling great. I felt the lump in my armpit area, thought it was scar tissue from reconstructive surgery. From when I was diagnosed I began Oil three weeks later and chemotherapy two weeks after that."

"[After taking Cannabis] I sleep like a baby, I feel healthy. I have energy because I'm always rested. I feel strong. I feel happy and brave. I use Cannabis Oil every night before bed. It's my life now, because it gave me my life back for me and my family. My blood work is perfect. **December 17th will be two years of being cancer-free**.

The Cannabis Oil is made from the strain Lavender Kush, which tested at 80% THC. I also mixed some of the Cannabis Oil with coconut oil on my neck at night. Those tumours went away in five weeks so I felt that nine grains of rice worth each night, plus the topical application, was good and working for me.

[The oil is] taken under the tongue and I used it topically on my neck as I had very large tumours growing from my collar bone towards the brain stem. I started with [the size of] a grain of rice, and increased to another grain every 4-

15

5 days. I got up to nine grains of rice per night and I felt that it was enough for me."

"The choice to use Cannabis Oil was an amazing opportunity to have. [...] It saved my life. I think I would have died for sure like the doctors told us if I had not done the Oil."

Source: www.cannabisoilsuccessstories.com/breast-cancer---triple-negative---stage-4.html

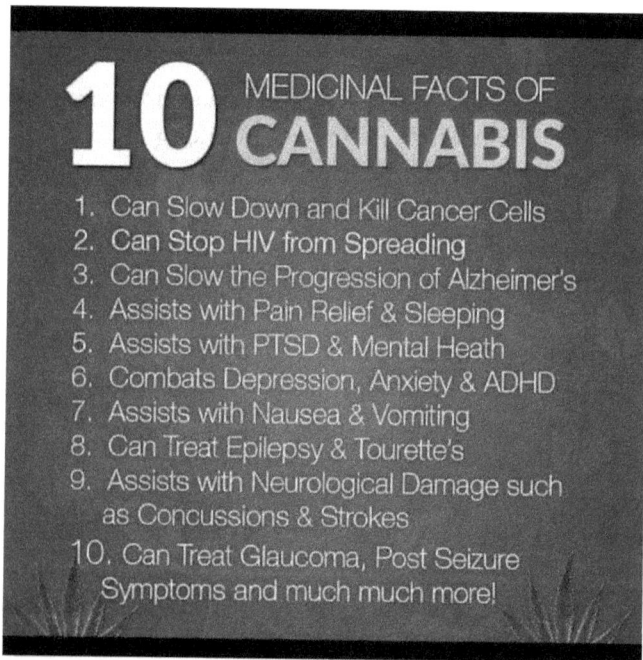

10 MEDICINAL FACTS OF CANNABIS

1. Can Slow Down and Kill Cancer Cells
2. Can Stop HIV from Spreading
3. Can Slow the Progression of Alzheimer's
4. Assists with Pain Relief & Sleeping
5. Assists with PTSD & Mental Heath
6. Combats Depression, Anxiety & ADHD
7. Assists with Nausea & Vomiting
8. Can Treat Epilepsy & Tourette's
9. Assists with Neurological Damage such as Concussions & Strokes
10. Can Treat Glaucoma, Post Seizure Symptoms and much much more!

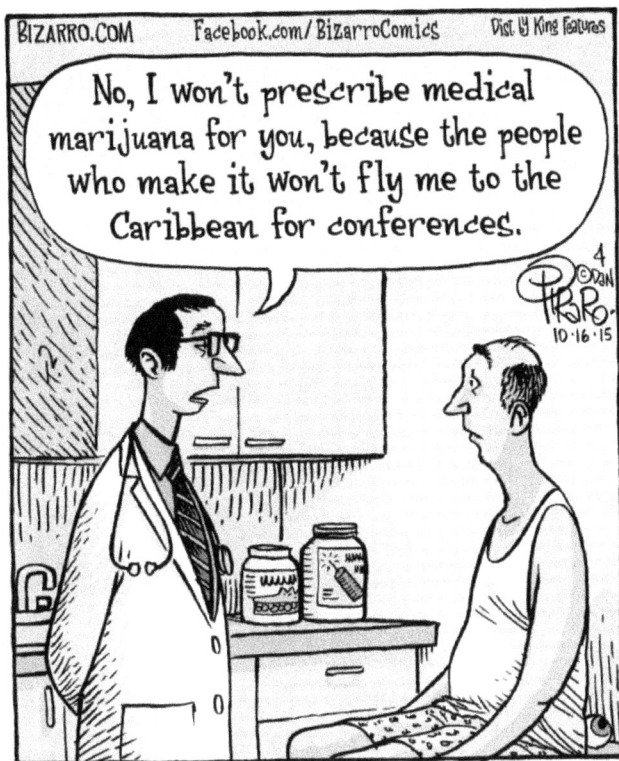

Is Western Medicine Afraid of Cannabis?

"What if I told you your own medical profession holds back cures, refuses to approve alternative medicines and procedures because they threaten the very structure of the "healing" profession? Doctors in the West deny the healing efficacies of doctors in the East because to accept them, to admit that certain alternate modalities might just provide some healing, would be to tear at the very fabric of the institution as it has structured itself. ... because to those institutions it's a matter of survival. The profession doesn't do this because it is evil. It does it because it is scared."

Neale Donald Walsch, *Conversations with God*

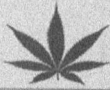

Can Industrial Cannabis (Hemp) Save The World?

CHAPTER 2

Healing From Colon Cancer

Colon cancer is the third most commonly diagnosed cancer and numbers are rising. In this chapter, I share five incredible stories of people who have cured their colon cancer using Cannabis oil.

Case Study #4: David Hibbitt Beats Terminal Colon Cancer After Chemo Failed

"A 33-year-old U.K. father, David Hibbitt, cured what doctors deemed a 'terminal' case of colon cancer with cannabis oil after radiation, chemotherapy and surgery all failed him. He had initially rejected the idea, but after being told he had just 18 months left to live, he was willing to try anything."

"Hibbitt used a high-potency variety known as Phoenix Tears and is now cancer-free. He also said that his 'pain just seemed to disappear'."

"Initially opting for chemotherapy, radiation *and* surgery – and watching this all fail – Hibbitt decided to take control of his own health by researching his condition online. When he came upon information outlining cannabis oil as a viable treatment alternative, he decided to give it a go with amazing results."

"According to the *Daily Mail Online*, Hibbitt went the cannabis route as a last-ditch effort when all else failed, and it turned out to be the best decision he could have made. As of January, **medical scans show that Hibbitt is completely cancer-free,** all thanks to the concentrated cannabis oil that he took from small vials provided by a local dealer."

"Friends had told me about cannabis oil and I dismissed it at first," Hibbitt explains, "I've never been into drugs. But in February last year I was told I only had 18 months to live, and I felt I had to try everything I could. I felt like chemo was killing me and I had nothing to lose. I couldn't accept I was going to die."

Understandably hesitant due to the stigma that still surrounds this powerful healing plant, Hibbitt thought long and hard about his options before concluding that cannabis was worth a go, especially in light of the health damage he'd already undergone as a result of invasive chemotherapy.

He contacted a local manufacturer of high-potency cannabis oil, a therapeutic grade of which is commonly referred to as 'Phoenix Tears' and was able to procure the amount he would need for treatment. The result, he says, is evident in his now-clean bill of health.

"The pain just seemed to disappear, and it seems to have done the job. I just want to make other people aware that there are other options out there."

One would think that Hibbitt's amazing recovery from advanced-stage bowel cancer using natural cannabis oil would be the subject of international headlines, with health officials everywhere scrambling to end prohibition in order to allow people to grow and use their own healing medicines for minimal cost compared to chemotherapy and radiation. But this is far from what's actually happening.

Like with most other natural cancer treatments, nearly *all* of which are outlawed in the U.S., cannabis oil is still regarded as "unproven" or even "dangerous" by the establishment, which would rather that cancer patients undergo poisoning than consume a healing plant with literally dozens of healing compounds.

"We know that cannabinoids – the active chemicals found in cannabis – can have a range of different effects on cancer cells grown in the lab and animal tumours," admits Dr. Kat Arney from Cancer Research U.K., at the same time citing the excuse that there "isn't good evidence from clinical trials" to prove that these compounds actually help cancer patients. But the proof is in the patients who've successfully used it and experienced miraculous healing from it."

Source: www.dailymail.co.uk

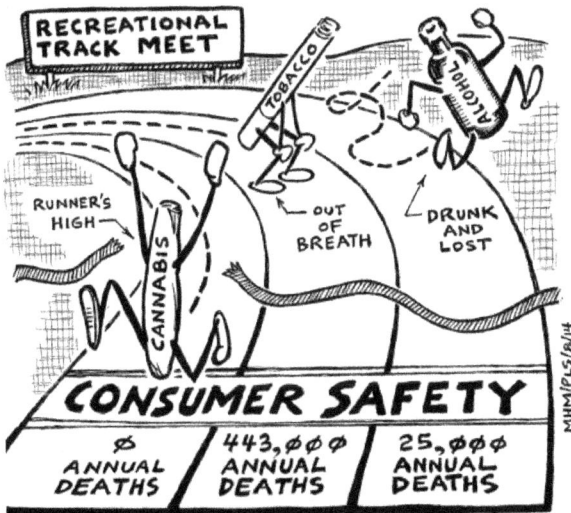

Case Study #5: Corrie Yelland Told
She Had 4 Months To Live

"Hi, My name's Corrie Yelland. I'm 55 years old. In May of 2007, I had a heart attack and subsequently had a double bypass. As a result of the heart surgery, for 4 plus years I have been plagued with chronic debilitating pain from a maligned sternum and post sternotomy neuralgia syndrome. I was ingesting copious amounts of various pain killers 24/7. They barely touched the pain. I spent my days in agony, waiting for evening so I could try to sleep. I took sleeping pills nightly in a futile attempt to escape the hell I was going through and failed miserably. Within 2 hours of taking the pills, I would awake in agony.

Fast forward to July of 2011. Already coping with two spots of skin cancer on my collar bone, I was stunned when I was diagnosed with Anal Canal Cancer (this is the same cancer that took Farrah Fawcett's life). Following two surgeries, the doctor told me they did not get all the cancer and I would have to endure a regime of radiation treatments. I started researching what this would entail and attended an intake meeting at the Cancer Clinic. I was informed that "this is the worst area of the body to radiate, the radiation beam would hit both my coccyx and pubic bone potentially causing permanent damage." They would try not to hit my spine.

Additionally, I would suffer 2nd and 3rd degree burns vaginally, rectally, across my buttocks, as well as my entire "nether regions", and there was a "good possibility" both my vagina and rectum would fuse shut from the burns and there would be subsequent scaring.

The list of both short and long-term side effects was endless and horrendous, but you get the gist. I told the doctor I needed time to think about it. His response was hostile, as he told me I had 2-4 months, possibly 6 to live. **He murmured something about a "death wish" and walked out.**

One day someone sent me Rick Simpson's video, 'Run from the Cure'. It took me days to get around to watching it, but when I did I was blown away. Here was this man, a seemingly super straight, small-town Nova Scotian, talking about these amazing results he had seen in himself and other people taking Cannabis and curing themselves of a myriad of diseases including end stage cancers.

After hearing what Rick had to say, and watching the testimonials in the video, I was feeling some hope for the first time. For 2 weeks I did nothing but research cannabis as a medicine. I was stunned by the sheer number of studies on Pub Med indicating that cannabis indeed has the capacity to heal. I started using cannabis 2 months ago as per Rick Simpson's protocol from his video. (He recommends starting out small, and slowly upping the dose so one's body becomes accustomed to it, without being high constantly. **I had huge hopes to cure my cancer and embarked on my fight to live.**

As well as ingesting the cannabis oil, I topically applied it to 2 spots of skin cancer on my collar bone. Within 48 hours, there were visible changes. **In just over a week, the 2 spots were completely gone.** Elated, I continued ingesting the oil, in hopes it would work on the other cancer attacking my body. Nothing prepared me for what happened next. **About 2 weeks into my regime, the pain in my sternum, as well as the nerve pain, had become almost non-existent.**

Never, in my wildest dreams, did I imagine I would be pain-free ever again. I was able to stand up straight, the jolting pain, so intense, ceased completely. I started to sleep through the night and stopped taking sleeping pills.

23

I saw one of my doctors a couple of weeks ago and was thrilled to hear **he believes there is a decrease in both the size and number of tumours.** I know in my heart it is only a matter of time before I will be completely cured. Even the most sceptical of my friends comment on the visible changes in me.

I have evolved from a pain wracked, hunched over, shuffling along individual, to a vibrant, high energy person. Even my complexion has improved. I get very emotional when I think of how far I've come. Not only has cannabis changed my life, **it is SAVING my life.**

When researching, I met a woman in Texas diagnosed with the same cancer that I have. Diagnosed at the same time, we felt fortunate to have found each other, as we were identical in every aspect (i.e. same age, same diagnostic procedure, same stage of the cancer with radiation recommended as treatment). She chose to have the radiation. I'm very sad to tell you she died 2 weeks ago as a result of infection from radiation burns. She left behind a husband and 12-year-old daughter.

At the end of May, I saw the doctor who first discovered my cancer. I was in the operating room for a non-related problem. At the time, I was told **he could no longer manually or visually detect any cancer.**

On September 20, 2012, I saw my specialist/surgeon, whom I had not seen for approximately 6 months. He examined me once, then a second time, and then a third time. My heart was pounding so loudly I could hear the whooshing in my ears. And then the news I had only dared to hope for. **"It's gone! I can't find anything at all. If it wasn't for the scar tissue I would never have known you had ever had cancer."**

Source: www.cannabiscure.info/corrie-yelland

Case Study #6: Gerry Says You Have Nothing To Lose And Everything To Gain By Using Cannabis Oil

"I was a 66-year-old male who was living in what I considered a normal healthy life with no major issues and maintained myself with a yearly flu shot and check-ups. My body functions were fine, and all seemed ok until I awoke one morning with awful stomach pain. Thinking it was appendix or hernia my wife rushed me to emergency. I had surgery about two hours later, August 15, 2012, to remove a massive tumour on my colon, along with 14 lymph nodes. One week later my insides broke open and poisoned me and that led to a second surgery.

Starting to feel better four days later, I was on my feet and slowly getting mobility back and I started to bleed out. Back for surgery number three and a day later had a mild heart attack. Shortly after that and after 33 days in ICU, I was discharged and toting an ostomy bag. The bag was with me eight months and a reversal surgery was done with no complications. The surgeon said cancer had not spread beyond the nodes. In spite of that they had marched me to the Cancer Clinic before discharge and started to discuss Chemotherapy and radiation as a "follow-up." Standard protocol they said. BULLSHIT said I! There will be no radiating my body or poisoning it with Chemo. The oncologist at the Cancer Clinic did not argue and outlined follow-ups every three months for a year, which entailed a CT Scan and blood work.

I sourced the material and produced the Cannabis Oil. Following all instructions for the extraction process I had the finished oil in syringes and started to ingest it twice a day, a tiny amount each time, and over a few days kept increasing the dose. I consumed a total of approx. 55 grams in about three-and-a-half months.

25

From there I started a small daily maintenance dose. I hit on Phoenix Tears and have not looked back.

After my fourth follow-up at the Cancer Clinic **in May of 2013 they stated that the CT Scan does NOT show anything that would indicate the presence of CANCER.** The blood work showed CEA level at 1.40, down again over the three months, but what the heck, everyone has a cancer cell or two in them. They consider anything 5+ to cause concern.

Follow-up to the above: CT and blood work in April 2014 after no testing for one year. **Doctor says my blood is clean and, quote "Gerry, your colon is SPOTLESS."** At the time of this last check-up, I had been ingesting between 3/4 to a gram daily. I feel in great shape. I sleep like a baby-without the waking up crying every hour. To anyone suffering now from cancer I suggest you do the same. You have NOTHING to lose and everything to gain."

Source: www.cannabisoilsuccessstories.com/colon-cancer--71-yo-male.html

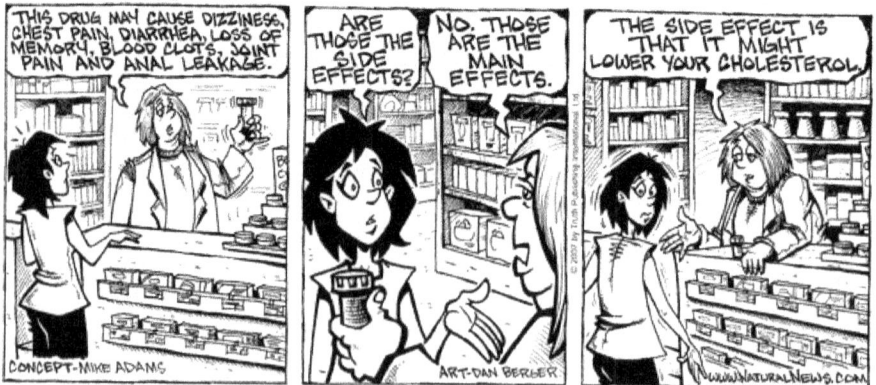

Thanks to Mike Adams and www.NaturalNews.com for the cartoon above.

Case Study #7: Lindsey From Cape Town Heals From Colon Cancer in 48 Days

"My name is Lindsey, and I live in Cape Town, South Africa. On August 12, 2011 my life changed forever. I had been to the doctor three times before about experiencing pain in my lower abdomen. He did the usual urine and blood test and announced it was a bladder infection. Weeks of antibiotics later, I was sicker than ever.

That morning, I woke with the most excruciating pain I had ever experienced. I could barely walk. Deep inside me, I knew it was something terrible.

My now husband, Brett, took me to another doctor who remarked, "Yes, I can definitely feel something in there, you need to go for an ultrasound," which confirmed an ovarian cyst, about 9cm in diameter, which had twisted on itself and was "causing chaos in my abdomen" - quoting the radiologist.

The gynaecologist, a sweet young woman, assured me everything would be okay, and I had surgery an hour later to remove the rogue ovary. **Waking up from that operation and hearing the news confirmed my biggest fear.** Apparently, while in the process of removing my ovary and cyst, they noticed something wrong with my colon, but closed me up anyway. I really don't understand what happened there. But after that operation, my colon and bladder had been punctured.

What follows is just too horrible to talk about, but slowly my body was becoming septic… and then, they sent me home. I'm sure it had nothing to do with the fact that I was a private patient. My gynaecologist bless her, in her good conscience, used her contacts to get a surgeon to operate at another much cheaper hospital, and a day later, I was in the ward waiting.

27

On the 25th of August 2011, I went in to surgery for the repair of my bladder and colon, and the temporary fitting of a colostomy bag. I found out later that the doctors were pleasantly surprised to see me alive the next morning; **the op was difficult, and they literally had to remove my insides and wash everything out with betadine!**

I surprised everyone with my quick recovery and the doctors were happy with my progress, just one final CT scan to make sure that I didn't have any remaining infection, and then I could go home. It was the 7th of September 2011. Brett had come to fetch me – we were waiting for a doctor to discharge me. I was already dressed when I watched his face and body movements as he walked towards me – I knew then. I was crying, maybe from relief, because I just knew there was something else.

The doctor blurted it out. I could see his eyes turning off, like they must be trained to say this without emotion. He spoke a whole lot of words I didn't hear, and then it came, and he apologized before he said it, too. Quote: "Sorry, you have cancer. You can go home and be with your family for the weekend [it was Friday], but you have to be back Monday. I'm giving you a weekend pass."

That evening, my daughter Kerry, my son Warren, Brett, and I spent time together talking. Life takes on a new perspective; you're completely alert, aware of every moment, taking it all in…taking in the value of the people in your life, and the precious memories you have. Then you realise that's actually all that counts. The support and love that came flooding in from family and friends was overwhelming. I have never, in my life, felt so loved and protected. What a blessing!

I went back to hospital on Monday, they monitored me (I had some 'mass' in my abdomen they were worried about), two days later, they discharged me with an appointment to the oncology ward in a few weeks. **The diagnosis – Stage 3 colon cancer.** They had cut out a tumour in my colon, but it was in my nodes, and there was spot on my liver. Only course of action was 6 months of chemotherapy, once a week, for 30 weeks, and to see what happens from there.

Chemo started on the 14th of October 2011. It sucked the life out of me… I could feel it slipping away. I found myself in limbo – trying to survive to the next week, to be strong enough for the chemo and the bouts of nausea and general yuckiness that zap your energy and leave you feeling morbidly depressed.

This time was a blur. I could barely work, I spent days and nights on the couch in a daze. Nausea was so bad, friends brought around weed, and I smoked some; it made things so much better. Not only could I enjoy food again, I slept better and generally felt a sense of wellbeing. I told my doctor about it and he said to take in as much as I could. He said he had done some research outside of his work and believed in its healing properties but was not in a position to give it to patients, or even to recommend it.

Halfway through my chemo (February 3, 2012 – 15 weeks in), I went for my halfway CT scan. My spirits were soaring! **I'd been living on a virtually organic vegetarian diet – berry smoothies, brown rice, greens, and salad** are what I live for. I'd been taking supplements every day for about 6 months: **vitamin C, green powder, hemp powder, spirulina, milk thistle, and bicarbonate soda.** I had no red meat or caffeine in my diet! I had every reason to believe I was clear and healthy and all I had to do was to convince them to reverse my op so that I could get rid of the colostomy bag. It didn't work out that way.

In the doctor's words, "There are now four spots on your liver, one on your kidney, and one on your gall bladder. But let's wait until we see the final report and I meet with the specialists to discuss." A week later, I went back. Well, **apparently this was damage from the chemo; the spot in my gall bladder was actually a 2.8 cm stone caused by the chemo**... the "spots" on my liver turned out to be lesions caused by the chemo...and kidney, turned out to be a cyst, again, caused by the chemo. Nothing more to say.

The chemo was causing more harm than good.

That day I made a life changing decision. I told the oncologist I wanted the chemo to stop and the remainder of my "treatment" to be an opportunity for me to heal myself holistically. She wasn't happy but gave me an appointment for the 23rd of May 2012. She said they would still follow protocol and treat me, even if I didn't take the chemo. I wondered whether she didn't worry too much because she probably believed I wouldn't be alive on the 23rd of May.

Around that time, I met some interesting people on Facebook **who had a lot to say about cannabis oil curing cancer.** I did all the research I could do and could only come up with positive things about the plant. The testimonials of people who had been cured were incredible. I can't mention names, but I wrote on the wall of one of the groups that were fighting to legalize cannabis, asking if anyone knew where I could get my hands on some cannabis oil. I already knew about the benefits while on chemo.

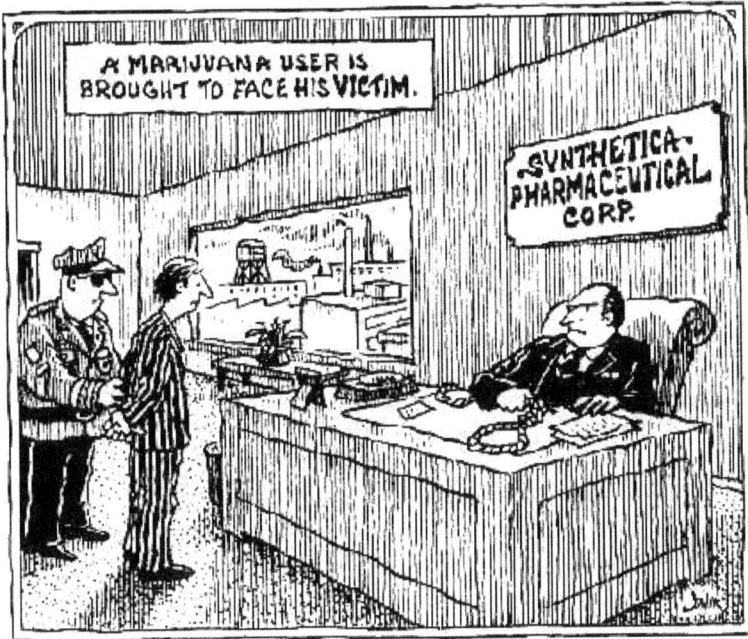

A few days later, the universe hooked me up with just the right person – and within days I was sorted. I paid R7200 ($900) for 6 syringes for the full dose needed to ingest to kill the cancer, which was 6 syringes full.

Cannabis is very strong, and the idea is to build up the daily dose over time. One dose is a drop on your finger, about the size of "half a grain of rice." The syringe is the easiest way to store and produce one drop of oil at a time. I took all 6 syringes, which totalled 18 grams, in 46 days. Most people take about 90 days.

There are loads of sites about cannabis oil, one of the best is Phoenix Tears, if you are looking for more information on the subject. I started my new treatment on the day I walked out of the hospital, declaring my 'independence'.

March 19, 2012… It's the day before my birthday… what a strange lap around the sun it's been. The past 12 months saw huge relationship lessons, health lessons, and, perhaps even more important, spiritual lessons. **It's Day 39 on the treatment and all is good...** even better than good. My eating (through research and experimentation) has become pretty much standard:

- ☐ Morning upon waking: 1 glass of water at room temperature with lemon juice (preferable organic)
- ☐ Breakfast: Strawberries, blueberries, raspberries, black grapes (Boiled egg on toast on weekends, or oats)
- ☐ Lunch: Salad: Avocado, rocket, spinach, celery, cucumber, kale (and variations thereof)
- ☐ Supper: Grilled fish or chicken with brown rice and/or salad.
- ☐ Every day: 8 glasses of water, rooibos (red tea), or chai tea (And the occasional glass of red or white wine in the evening, and/or dark chocolate)
- ☐ Supplements: Organic Grass Mix, Organic Seaweed Mix, Chlorella, Spirulina, Vitamin C, Organic Milk Thistle, Organic Dandelion, Sodium Bicarbonate (1 teaspoon in warm water every night before bed).

March 28, 2012... I'm at the hospital to see the oncologist and the surgeons who did my operation, to ask for them to schedule my "reversal" operation. I underwent a whole range of tests and scans and met later in the afternoon with four doctors present. **There is no sign of any cancer in my body!!**

What I have realized through this experience is **only I am responsible for my health and it's up to me to heal my body...no doctor can do that.** And no one knows what's best for me, but me! My cancer diagnosis was a true blessing. It facilitated a change within me on every level: emotionally, physically, mentally, and spiritually. It formed an unbreakable bond of love and support with my husband. I've become brave and confident in my own power to heal myself. This is truly the biggest blessing and I really want to help inspire others to do the same."

Source: http://communitybasedispensary.org/lindsey-cures-colon-cancer-with-cannabis-in-48-days

Case Study #8: John Gabriel Says Cannabis Oil Cured His Stage III Colon Cancer

"My name is John Gabriel. I was diagnosed with Stage III Colon Cancer, rapidly spreading through my body. I was told that I needed to have surgery, and that I would need a colostomy bag. I had chemo and radiation for about three weeks, which shrunk the tumour for it to be removed by operation. I didn't want that operation, and I informed my surgeon that I would not have it. Of course, she thought I was nuts. But I stuck to my guns, and strangely enough, the surgeon agreed with me.

She said "when the cancer comes back..." (It wasn't a case of "IF" it came back, but when!). She said when the cancer comes back [after the chemotherapy] there will be more cutting, more chemo, more radiation, and then you end up in crutches, and then in a wheelchair, and then on your deathbed. And these are the words she used.

It's really not a nice way to go. Because there is no painkillers for this. So that was all very, very bad news.

I found out through the grapevine about Cannabis oil. And I heard that it cured Cancer, but I didn't believe that. But there was still a hope attached to that... I found all kinds of testimonials about it on YouTube, the ability of cannabis to kill cancer...

Within 2 months, my cancer was completely gone. To the astonishment of my surgeon and all related personnel dealing with my cancer, such as the oncologist.

Radiation and chemotherapy are both cancerogenic. They cause cancer. **Had I listened to the medical team, I would have had my colon cut out**, I would be wearing a colostomy bag, and I would be on drugs... all kinds of them... to relieve the pain, I suppose, while Big Pharma would be making money off of this barbaric treatment."

Source: https://www.youtube.com/watch?v=vyCV4S2XvjI

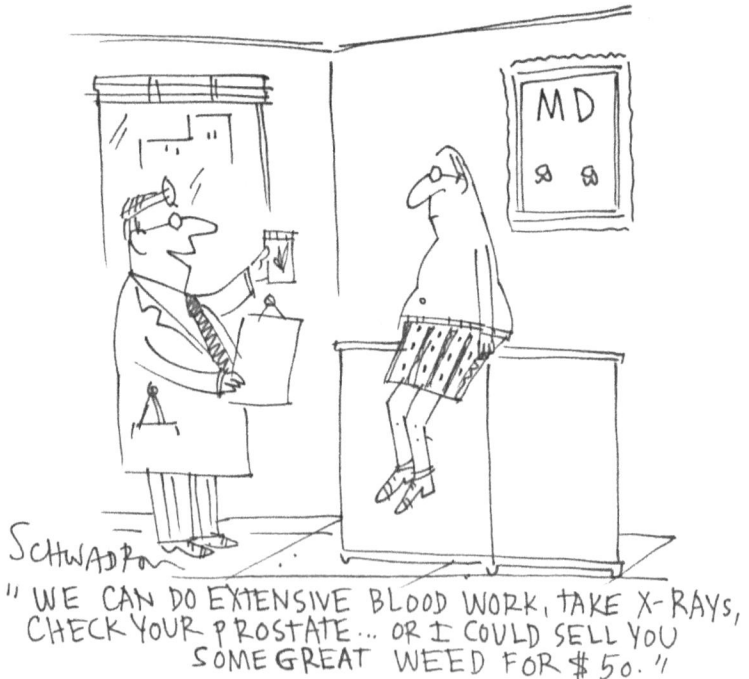

" WE CAN DO EXTENSIVE BLOOD WORK, TAKE X-RAYS, CHECK YOUR PROSTATE... OR I COULD SELL YOU SOME GREAT WEED FOR $50. "

CHAPTER 3

Healing From Lung Cancer

For many, a diagnosis of lung cancer can feel like a death sentence. But for the following four people, it was far from it.

Case Study #9: Sharon Kelly Diagnosed With Stage IV Lung Cancer, Told She Has 9 Months To Live

"Sharon Kelly is an Australian woman who was diagnosed with Stage IV non-small cell lung cancer on January 17th, 2014. Cancer had been found in various areas including her left lung and three lymph nodes.

The 5-year survival rate for lung cancer is only 1%. Treatment usually consists of chemotherapy and radiation to initially shrink tumours, then surgery to remove them. Chemotherapy offers virtually no hope of total remission. Kelly's situation looked dire.

Kelly initially had two intravenous chemotherapy treatments, and then was switched to an oral chemotherapeutic drug called Tarceva. Kelly's life expectancy was between 6 and 9 months.

Kelly did her own research and discovered that cannabis oil may be able to completely eliminate her cancer. For years, scientific studies and anecdotal evidence have supported the effectiveness of cannabis extracts for lung cancer treatment.

Not wasting time, she added the cannabis oil to her traditional therapy in February 2014. For a short time, she also directly juiced raw cannabis leaf, which can enhance the effectiveness of cannabis oil by supporting it with raw cannabis nutrients. To avoid psycho-activity and increase dosage, Kelly also began taking cannabis oil through suppositories.

Her dramatic turnaround defied doctors' predictions and medical statistics. Since her success, Kelly has helped thousands of people through her story and direct communications with other patients."

"Her cannabis treatment started in May 20, 2014, and her cancer was gone by Sept. 3, 2014. Within three months, her cannabis oil treatment cured her stage IV lung cancer!"

Source:www.naturalnews.com/047924_lung_cancer_cannabis_oil_medical_marijuana.html and https://illegallyhealed.com/sharon-kelly

Case Study #10: 60-Year-Old Man Cured of Lung Cancer

"When my dad was diagnosed in September, my family and I were devastated. He's 60 years old, always worked hard, golfed every week, and up until late July, never had any symptoms. In late July, he began having severe headaches. He went to the doctor and had an MRI. That's when they found a brain tumour. He was referred to a neurologist who, after reviewing the MRI, saw a second brain tumour. BOTH tumours we're initially diagnosed as benign. They explained that they would b able to remove one, but not the other. It wasn't imperative though, because it was benign and just something to watch.

Within a few weeks, my father had the surgery to remove the one that could be removed. Obviously, my family and I were nervous and scared, but extremely thankful there was no cancer. When the surgery was completed, the neurosurgeon met my family and I in the waiting room. He seemed a bit nervous and looked a little baffled. That's when he explained that he was unable to remove the whole tumour as it had begun to attach itself to surrounding tissue and that he now believed this to be cancerous, but not brain cancer. He ordered a full body scan to be done within a week or so. On September 15, 2016, he told my dad that **they found an 8-inch mass on his lung.** The scan also revealed Mets to the lymph node, liver, spine and they also found a third one on the brain. My dad was diagnosed with stage IV Non-Small Cell Lung Cancer.

No medications were being taken prior to Cannabis. When he was diagnosed, I immediately started researching and that's when I discovered CBD & THC oils. I started making the oil and giving it to him. He began chemo treatments at about same time. He had six sessions of Carboplatin.

We started THC Oil and CBD Oil in mid-October. At first, it was about a drop of THC Oil three times a day. Much more CBD Oil, probably one dropper full, three times a day. He is now taking about 18 drops of the THC Oil, three times a day and the CBD Oil- two droppers full, three times a day under the tongue.

He started gaining weight within a month. It is imperative to use both THC and CBD Oils. CBD Oil can be bought online. The THC Oil has to be made. Google "How to make THC Oil for cancer". […] In addition, **I have him vaping THC Oil at least 2-3 times a day. It's especially helpful with lung cancer.**

There is scientific evidence proving Cannabis causes programmed cell death to cancerous cells, thus resulting in not only killing the cancer, but preventing it from spreading. As of March 16, 2017, he has gained back about 20 pounds (he initially lost 35). **The body scan results show significant shrinkage of ALL tumours.** Lung, lymph, liver and spine. The lung tumour went from 8cm to 2cm. All others are smaller than 2cm. **The brain MRI showed NO tumours. They are gone."**

Source: www.cannabisoilsuccessstories.com/non-small-cell-lung-cancer---stage-iv--60-yo-male.html

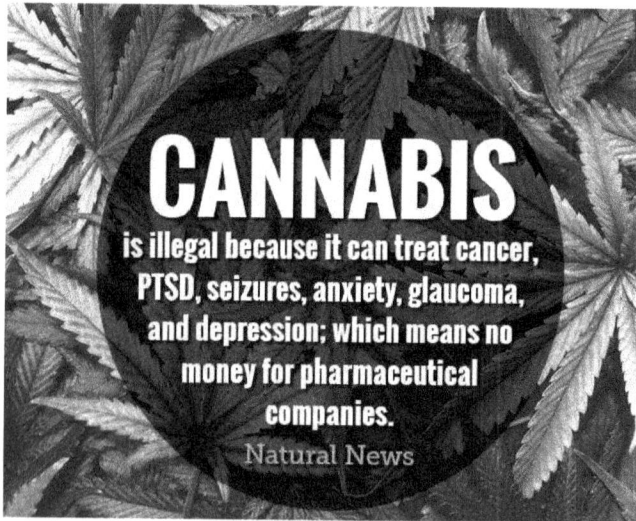

Case Study #11: Mitch Johnson's Remarkable Story

"Mitch Johnson is a Utah resident with 30 years of contracting experience. He has worked hard and dealt with a lot in his life, including childhood abuse and trauma. Using a combination of modern techniques and cannabis, he has also overcome cancer twice.

In 2003, Mitch was diagnosed with leiomyosarcoma, an especially rare type of soft tissue cancer that can appear nearly anywhere in the body. For Mitch, it was his left testicle, which was removed to eliminate the cancer. Doctors warned him the cancer could return.

Indeed, in September 2013, a chest X-ray revealed the cancer had returned with a 1.5cm tumour in his left lung and **a shotgun pattern of small tumours in his right lung.** Mitch had been prompted to get this X-ray because he was coughing up blood, although the cause of this bleeding turned out to be a sinus infection rather than the cancer.

Mitch was aware of the research surrounding the medical benefits of cannabis, such as fighting cancer. (A 2007 Harvard study shows tetrahydrocannabinol (THC) can shrink lung tumours in animals. THC, along with cannabidiol (CBD), also help the body's own immune system destroy lung cancer cells).

Within a week of being diagnosed, Mitch started smoking cannabis in the hopes it would fight his cancer. At the end of October, he procured cannabis oil in the form of 'Trippy Stix', vaporizers with pre-loaded cannabis oil. In addition to smoking cannabis and vaporizing oil, he ingested edibles when possible.

Mitch made nutritional changes like cutting out soft drinks and mostly eating vegetarian meals. He also took Essiac tea and Tru-Pine (other alternative anti-cancer treatments), and began exercising more.

In June 2014, Mitch had surgery to remove a third of the lower left lobe of his lung. A subsequent X-ray revealed that **eight of the nine tumours on his right lung were gone.** The doctors didn't know how to explain this and said he was a 'unique case'. Also unique is the fact Mitch has not been sick for one day in the past 18 months, and lung tests show he is blowing at 125% of normal.

Besides the potential direct anti-cancer effect, cannabis has been amazing for Mitch's mental well-being. Every time he thought about dying and got anxious, he would take a hit and stop worrying within three minutes. This anxiolytic effect also helped Mitch deal with issues related to past abuse and his divorce. Although Mitch is not 100% cancer free, he is hopeful that with more time and hopefully a true course of extract treatment, he will regain perfect health."

Source: https://illegallyhealed.com/stopping-lung-cancer-with-modern-and-alternative-treatments

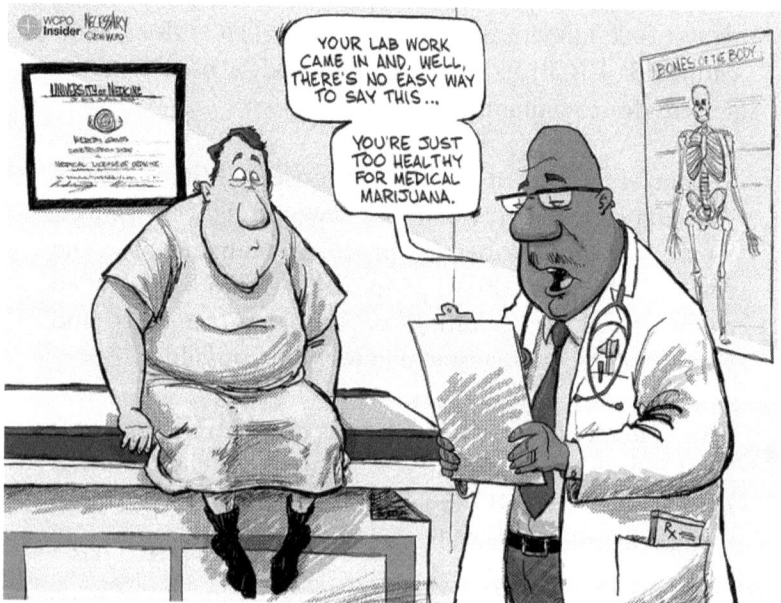

"Cartoon by Kevin Necessary, courtesy of WCPO/E.W. Scripps Co."

CHAPTER 4

Healing From Skin Cancer, Melanomas, and Carcinomas

In this chapter, I share six remarkable stories of individuals who have turned to cannabis extracts to treat their skin cancers and their individual experiences using this natural alternative as a treatment.

Case Study #12: Rick Simpson's Skin Cancer Vanishes Thanks To Cannabis Oil

"In 2003 Rick was diagnosed with basal cell carcinoma skin cancer. He had 3 spots of cancer on his body; two on his face and one on his neck.

After not having much luck with surgery Rick decided to try something different. For almost a year Rick had been extracting the oil from the cannabis plant and ingesting it orally. He had been taking the oil for other health reasons, but the cancer diagnosis gave him an idea. He remembered a radio headline that stated that the University of Virginia had found the THC cannabinoid in cannabis could kill cancer in mice.

He figured that if it kills cancer in mice it would kill his cancer, too. Rick applied the oil to some bandages and put them on the skin cancer. **After 4 days, to Rick's surprise the cancer was gone.** His cannabis oil had cured his cancer.

Rick tried to tell his doctors but they wouldn't listen. He even went to the cancer organizations and tried to get their help but nobody wanted anything to do with his discovery. At that point Rick took matters into his own hands. He started growing cannabis on his own land and producing his own cannabis oil. He gave the oil away for free to anyone who needed it. Even after having his home raided multiple times and having over 2600 cannabis plants cut down and taken by the RCMP, he continued to produce the oil and help others.

In 2008 Rick put out a documentary on YouTube called Run From The Cure. This documentary has been viewed millions of times worldwide and has helped millions of people. It's now been over 10 years since Rick began his journey. **Rick has healed over 5,000 people** with this amazing oil, not to mention the countless others all over the world who have heard his story."

Source: www.cureyourowncancer.org/rick-simpson.html

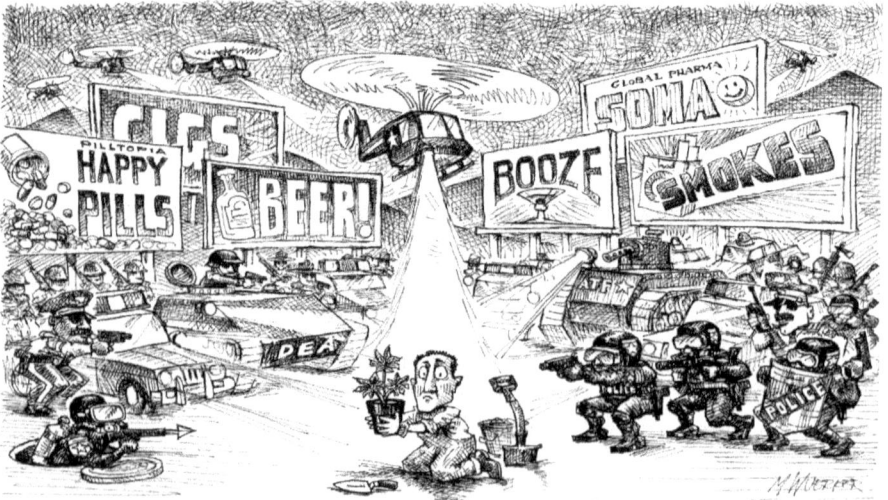

Case Study #13: Skin Cancer Cleared Up with Cannabis Oil

"[I was diagnosed with] Skin cancer. I went to a Dermatologist for confirmation, although I would not let them do a biopsy so there is no "official" diagnosis. I had a spot on my hip, that appeared all of the sudden. It had different colours, irregular shape, all the markings of melanoma. It was the size of maybe a butter bean. It was raised up off skin. I also had a flat spot on my arm that always seemed to be irritated, especially when it got sun. It became inflamed, and crusty. The Dermatologist said my arm spot was definitely either squamous or basal carcinoma and from just looking at my hip spot, it most definitely looked like melanoma. His advice was to remove them asap. I said I would think about it and left. He was very short with me, almost angry.

I had no intention of doing biopsies on either. It is my belief, from all I have researched and also experienced with others, that once you start cutting into the cancer, it spreads. Anyone I know who has had skin cancer cut out is continuously going to the doctor to have it cut out. I wanted to try some natural methods first.

The first thing I tried was Frankincense Oil on the spot on my hip. I applied it a minimum of twice a day. The spot shrank by at least 50% in a few weeks' time. During this time, I heard about the Cannabis Oil and began to produce my own. I then used the Cannabis Oil on the spot on my arm, covered with a band-aid, changed out with fresh oil each day for six weeks. I may have used it longer than necessary because in the beginning it looked like a raw, open blister and looked that way for all those weeks, mainly I think because the air did not get to it. I quit applying the Cannabis Oil because my arm became itchy and red, almost like hives all around the spot.

43

After not applying the oil and letting it go without a band-aid, **it scabbed over and cleared up and it is gone** and has not given me another bit of trouble. I also applied it to my spot on my hip, it reduced it in size further; it is still about half the size of an eraser and is very light coloured and has not changed in months. I may do another treatment with the oil on it, not sure. I am not convinced it is/was melanoma. From my research it appears it could have just been a benign vascular growth. Either way I believe that **the Cannabis Oil made a huge difference with both spots.**

I made my own Full Extract Cannabis Oil using 100-proof alcohol. Personally, I believe if there is a way to use a natural God-given plant, herb to heal and help ourselves it is always far better than a synthetic drug."

Source: www.cannabisoilsuccessstories.com/skin-cancer.html

Case Study #14: Mike McShane's Miraculous Recovery From Skin Cancer

"Mike McShane has endured five bouts of Squamous cell carcinoma cancer. He's spent a million dollars and has been treated with radiation therapy, chemotherapy and surgery by this team of doctors at the Detroit Medical Center. Today, he believes the invasive treatments were unnecessary. He says he's cured his latest bout with the disease using a highly concentrated form of cannabis oil.

Three years ago, I wouldn't have believed the so-called, "healing properties of cannabis," but not today. Not with 51-year-old McShane sitting across from me, grinning through the smoke and nodding his head. He's a rapt audience of one, sitting in the front pew in the church of healing.

25 years ago, McShane was diagnosed with HIV. This was the late 80's, when nothing was known about the disease. **Doctors gave you an immediate death sentence.**

"The opportunistic diseases that kill you with HIV are cancer and pneumonia," he says, "I went in with breathing problems and asking what time I was leaving. They said, 'you'll be lucky if you get out of here in two weeks alive.'"

"I felt a wheelchair bump me in the back of the legs, and heard, 'sit down sir,' then they wheeled me into an ICU isolated unit. Everybody had space suits on. Anyone who came into that room was dressed up like they were landing on the moon or ready to fight chemical warfare. They looked like Robby the Robot coming at me."

"There they were, my caregivers, all suited up and I'm thinking, 'man I must be super messed up'."

The doctor came in and told McShane, "I'll give you six months to live. Do you have any questions?"

"He was really sarcastic," McShane says, adding that at that time, HIV was 'The Gay' disease. "I was shaking and thinking what the hell? It was unbelievable."

McShane's first bout with cancer occurred a few years later. His doctors cut a wedge out of his lip. Soon after, he noticed a lump in his neck. He underwent radical neck surgery that removed part of his jugular vein. He also underwent radiation treatment.

"By the time they were done I couldn't talk, plus they cut the nerve in my neck. I had to learn how to talk again. The radiation they used on me was so strong it burned my throat."

A few years after the neck dissection, McShane experienced colon cancer, which resulted in surgery and chemotherapy. "The colon cancer was a pain in the ass," he laughs, "but it wasn't anything like the neck surgery."

After the colon issue McShane had a major outbreak of cancer in four areas on his face. They performed surgery on his forehead, both lips and cheek in a surgical suite, using local anaesthetic while McShane was awake. He says he could feel everything and asked for more anaesthesia.

The doctor would first remove tissue, then send it to a nearby lab for testing while McShane waited in the chair. He repeated this process until all the cancer was gone. **By then, he had removed a substantial amount of Michael McShane's face.**

He was rushed out through the back of the clinic. "I walked in looking normal and now it looked like a pipe bomb went off in my face," he says, "From a marketing perspective, they had me go out the back door."

After eight hours of reconstructive surgery, and another six procedures for scar revisions and lip clefts, McShane's oncology procedure was deemed successful.

In June of 2011, the cancer on his face returned, growing back in the same places where it had been surgically removed. By then he was growing marijuana, acting as a caregiver under the Medical Marihuana Act. McShane recalls a powerful, dawning moment of learning that marijuana cured cancer.

"There I was in the basement, with the plants growing, and the lights and fans humming. I couldn't believe it. The thought of curing my cancer with this oil was almost too much."

"I got Simpson oil and started putting it on and after ten days, ten days I saw it. **The cancer started to break up before my eyes.** It looked like a big white callous, and it started to fragment and break up. I was crying. It was unbelievable."

He called his Dermatologist, told him the cancer was back and that he was treating it with marijuana. McShane leaps from his chair in my office and starts dancing around, laughing. "Here I am, in my basement, with a 9th grade education and I'm healing my cancer, and I'm saying, 'I'm not going to spend 40 grand with you!'"

He went to his doctor's office. "You've got cancer on your face," he told McShane.

"I know," he responded. "That's the reason I'm here. I want you to put it in my chart and note it because when I come back I don't think it'll be here. It's going to be gone because I'm using this marijuana oil."

His doctor told him, "Well ok, but get to Dermatology immediately. That's cancer." McShane didn't go to Dermatology. He continued using the oil and the cancer started to lose the battle very quickly. It took about three months to reach the underneath layer of live skin. During that time, he went to see his doctor about four times who said he could see things were getting better.

When McShane went to see his doctor for his last visit, he expected him to proclaim a miracle, **"He took a look at my face and was amazed, but made no comments whatsoever, as if he really didn't know what to do.** I think he got a phone call from Newman and had been 'talked to' because when he came into to look at me it was more of a political thing than a doctor's exam."

"I said to him, 'Normally at this point you'd pull a knife on me. Is there any cause for concern?' and he said, 'No. You look great.' He asked to follow up at 16 weeks."

"He wasn't being a doctor. He was protecting the medical industry. **It was the weirdest thing that's ever happened to me. I thought we'd be on Fox news and we'd have a parade down Woodward.**"

"With cancer it's a real fear-based system, a war-based mentality, fueled by the fear of cancer and dying and the trilogy of the whole thing is your insurance; that's what makes it all work. I've been diagnosed and cut on within hours. It's all about coming at you with nuclear weapons and knives."

"They have known that this cures cancer since 1974, and all these things that have happen to me have been since 1974, which means I wouldn't have had to do any of the things I've had to do with western medicine, or the costs that are associated with it, if they had allowed research on cannabis."

"**I cured myself in 90 days in my basement in Ferndale** as a patient, come on, we can get there in 10 years with labs. We did this! **The potheads did it with a rice cooker.**"

When I last saw Mike McShane, he was working on healing his HIV with an intense 90-day treatment of Simpson oil. **His cancer has not returned."**

Source: www.cureyourowncancer.org/michael-mcshanes-story-beating-squamous-cell-carcinoma-skin-cancer-with-cannabis-oil.html

Case Study #15: Basal Cell Carcinoma Treated with Cannabis

"Tumours emerge almost monthly since my initial diagnosis in 2004. Head, neck, back and legs. It's constant. Some tumours would develop and become so large so quickly, between my regular appointment times (every six months) with my former dermatologist, that excision was the only option. It was getting so bad, before I found Cannabis Oil, that I was seriously considering getting the chemotherapy cream. I felt I had no other choice.

I applied Cannabis Oil topically to tumours immediately upon detection, but the big breakthrough for Basal Cell Carcinoma (BCC) fighters, in my opinion, is using DMSO as an enhanced delivery agent for Cannabis Oil. I wholeheartedly believe that the combination of DMSO (applied before the cannabis oil) and Cannabis oil helps to eradicate tumours much faster than Cannabis Oil by itself. From what I have read BCC sufferers get good results with Cannabis Oil except for those whose skin still covers their tumours. **I think DMSO is what these fighters need to get the oil through the skin and deep into the tumour.** And for those who successfully treat BCC with cannabis oil it can take months whereas I have experienced complete eradication, with no scarring, in weeks on a major tumour and eradication in one week for emerging tumours.

I am now healthy and happy, tumours are eradicated within a week of initial detection. It's amazing. No more visiting the dermatologist every six months. No more watching tumours develop."

Source: www.cannabisoilsuccessstories.com/basal-cell-carcinoma.html

Case Study #16: 57-Year-Old Woman Has Carcinoma Treated with Cannabis Extract

"I had a lump under my right jaw, in April 2014. After investigations, the doctor told me it wasn't cancer, it is a virus, the lump will grow for a while, and I have no reason to be concerned. He reassured me several times that it was not cancer.

I was very sick. I started having big digestive problems and I couldn't eat anything. My skin turned yellow-grey and I was constantly very tired. I was sweating during the nights.

[...] I started taking Cannabis Oil with 80% THC, Indica strain, three days after I got diagnosed [with cancer]. It relaxed me, helped me to sleep, increased my appetite. Cannabis Oil gave me peace of mind and helped me reconnect with myself. This was HUGE. **In a few days I began feeling like myself again**. No more fears of cancer or the surgery that had to come. After the surgery, it helped increase my appetite and helped me sleep.

Before Cannabis Oil, emotionally, I was a mess. The Oil put me back on track in days. I believe the oil healed my body and my mind. After the surgery I got pancreatitis, and all my internal organs were not functioning properly. I lost 20 pounds in one month. Pancreatitis is not only very painful, but makes you feel like you are going to die any minute. **I started taking Cannabis Oil with 60% CBD. In FOUR hours, my pain was gone**, and in one day my nausea was gone. My mind was more relaxed, without having that constant panic state anymore. I started healing but very slow."

Both oils I have make me very high. I take about one gram a month, maybe a bit more. I take CBD oil at least two hours away from the THC. I take as much as I can without getting very high, but I am very far from that *60 grams in 90 days* protocol.

Without cannabis oil I wouldn't be here. It gives me peace of mind. I can focus on healing, without fear. It gives me appetite. It healed my pancreatitis. It keeps the cancer cells under control. I will take it my whole life, and I will try to educate people about the benefits."

Source: www.cannabisoilsuccessstories.com/basal---squamous-cell-carcinoma--57-yo-female.html

Case Study #17: 30-Year-Old Woman In Remission From Stage 4 Melanoma Thanks To Cannabis

"[Before Cannabis extracts] I looked physically very healthy, but I was destroying my body with over-exercise (I was a marathon runner and Crossfit competitor but exercising 3+ hours a day on around 1000 calories a day) and alcohol. I was absolutely on the path to alcoholism and had tried AA. I was diagnosed with Von Willebrands Disease, which makes me very anaemic and makes menstrual cycles to be pretty darn awful. I was also on numerous medications for diagnosed anxiety, insomnia, ADHD.

[After Cannabis extracts]: **Cancer free! I've been in remission for a year and cannabis helped me get there.** Arguably more importantly, I also have absolutely zero desire to drink now. What an unintended consequence of cancer, but I'm clean and sober and happier than I've ever been! I was self-medicating with alcohol to control severe anxiety, insomnia, and ADHD. **Cannabis has allowed me to get off every single medication I was on before.** In fact, I can have a glass of wine at dinner and have absolutely zero desire to continue drinking. I've also joined a new company and

51

have been promoted because I'm a much better employee and leader now.

I used concentrated Cannabis Oil during treatment in conjunction with chemotherapy and radiation, but only in my last few months of treatment. Ultimately, THC worked better than pure CBD oils, and even then, I did much better with edibles and tinctures. My maintenance regimen now is 20mg CannaOil around 4PM, (THC-heavy strains, primarily Indicas, usually at 18% or higher with coconut oil) and tinctures (alcohol-based, I have a glycerin allergy!) another 30mg before bed. This looks like a teaspoon of oil on my salad at dinner, and half a tablespoon of Oil mixed into whatever before bed. I use tinctures mostly when traveling. I grow my own OR swap with others, and I make the tincture and CannaOil myself.

It's changed my life. Now I feel at peace. I like myself, I like who I've become. I'm an excellent wife, employee, cat mama, daughter, and I was not before Cannabis. I'm also alive! Life is good."

Source: www.cannabisoilsuccessstories.com/melanoma-stage-4--30-yo-female.html

"Twenty-five years in which I used prescribed drugs, and 33 years in which I have not used prescribed drugs, should make my belief that drugs are unnecessary and in most cases injurious, worth something to those who care to know the truth."

John H. Tilden, M.D. (1940)

CHAPTER 5

Healing From Stomach and Bowel Cancer

The testimonials I share in this chapter will shed some light on how those suffering with stomach cancer can benefit by using medicinal cannabis.

Case Study #18: Stage 4 Cancer in Stomach, Throat, and Pancreas; Bob was Given 2 Weeks to Live, Now in Remission

"In 2010 I accidentally stumbled upon the movie 'Run from the Cure' on YouTube. I was very sceptical when I initially heard that cannabis could cure cancer. Like everyone, I assumed that if there was a cure for cancer it wouldn't be kept quiet. After countless hours of watching videos and reading through articles and studies I began to change my opinion. There was so much science behind cannabis and its effects on cancer I couldn't believe it.

Since 1974 studies have shown that cannabis has anti-tumour effects. The results of the 1974 study, reported in an Aug. 18, 1974 Washington Post newspaper feature, were that cannabis's component, THC, "slowed the growth of lung cancers, breast cancers and a virus-induced leukaemia in laboratory mice, and prolonged their lives by as much as 36 percent."

In 1975 an article in the Journal of the National cancer institute titled 'Antineoplastic Activity of Cannabinoids', they reported that "Lewis lung adenocarcinoma growth was retarded by the oral administration of tetrahydrocannabinol (THC) and cannabinol (CBD). Mice treated for 20 consecutive days with THC and CBD had reduced primary tumour size."

In 1998, a research team at Madrid's Complutense University Led by Dr. Manuel Guzman discovered that THC can selectively induce programmed cell death in brain tumour cells without negatively impacting surrounding healthy cells. They reported in the March 2002 issue of 'Nature Medicine' they had destroyed incurable brain cancer tumours in rats by injecting them with THC. And in 2007, even Harvard Researchers found that compounds in cannabis cut the growth of lung cancer. There is also an organization called The SETH Group that showed compounds in cannabis can stop the growth of human glioblastoma multiforma (GBM) brain cancer cells. The SETH Group says, "No chemotherapy can match this nontoxic anti-cancer action." In 2012 a pair of scientists at California Pacific Medical Center in San Francisco found THC stops metastasis in many kinds of aggressive cancer. Those are just a few of the studies done that show the effects of cannabis on cancer.

So, over the next year and a half I began talking about this to pretty much anyone that would listen. In November 2011 all of that talking finally reached the right person. I was contacted by a man who was looking for help. This man wishes to remain anonymous, so I'll refer to him as Bob. Bob had stage 4 cancer in his stomach, throat and pancreas. Over the course of 6-8 weeks from when Bob was diagnosed, he became so sick he could no longer eat and he lost over 50lbs. He was actually supposed to be dead before thanksgiving and when I first talked to him he was given about 2 weeks to live.

Bob had been given radiation the month before he contacted me and he and his doctor were hopeful that would help. But instead of helping it seemed to make his cancer worse. So instead of trying to continue to help Bob, his doctor told him he was sorry, but the cancer had spread too much and there was nothing left to do for him. **Bob's doctor simply told him to go home and die.**

Bob has a son and when I first spoke with him he was so scared and sad about dying and leaving his son alone. Being a father myself I immediately felt for him and wanted to help. He asked me if I could help make the oil because he had no way of doing it alone, so I agreed to help him. **Within 2 days of our first conversation Bob was taking the cannabis oil.**

For the 8 weeks before Bob started to take the oil he wasn't able to keep real food down, so he lost about 50lbs. He was living on boost drinks and protein bars. Because the tumours in his body caused him so much pain he was unable to sleep. After his first dose of oil he was finally able to keep real food in his stomach and sleep soundly. He requested and ate 2 turkey sandwiches and a bowl of ice cream; he kept all of it down.

Bob went back to his doctor for an appointment 30 days after starting his treatment with cannabis oil. His doctor had scheduled the visit for 2 weeks after Bob was supposed to have been dead. Bob didn't tell his doctor he had started ingesting the oil and **when he went back his tumours had reduced by 20%.** His doctor was surprised at his progress, so he scheduled him for another appointment 30 days later.

On the 60-day appointment Bob would get his best news yet. **The cancer he had in his throat, stomach and pancreas had been reduced so significantly they considered him in 'remission'.** I would think that a doctor's first instinct would be to ask his patient what he has done differently to cause this change in his cancer, but that was not the case. Instead they offered him radiation for a second time. The second time though he decided not to take the treatment. He instead continued the cannabis oil treatment and is still alive today, cancer-free. It is a miracle of this God-given plant."

Case Study #19: Stage IV Gastroesophageal Cancer

"My boyfriend of 20 years was diagnosed with advanced stage four gastroesophageal cancer; tumour so large at the junction of the stomach and oesophagus that the camera for the endoscopy was nearly blocked. He did extensive chemo with 5-fu bottle tethered to his side… the tumour thrived. He then underwent total gastrectomy (complete stomach removal), lymphectomy (lymph nodes removed) splenectomy (spleen removed), partial removal of liver and half removal of oesophagus.

Daily radiation therapy was stopped after four weeks when he could no longer endure it. Cancer had returned and thrived again with the radiation given within only 6 months of his surgery. Another series of chemo was immediately scheduled, but we postponed it for a couple of weeks while we took what was thought would be our last chance to visit distant family.

I contacted Rick Simpson. As he instructed, I followed his recipe for making the oil exactly. I gave my boyfriend an amount equal to the size of a 1/4 grain of rice. Very strong stuff, but it's going to take something very strong to kick Cancer back.

Another CT scan was taken right before he was to start Chemo again, and another possible surgery scheduled. **The CT scan revealed No Evidence of Disease. His doctors were stunned**, and didn't know what to make of it. They said they've never seen anything like it.

My boyfriend is doing great, and August 2018 will be his 5-year mark. When he's not doing well, I give him the oil and he's fine again."

Source: www.cancercompass.com/message-board/message/all,136564,0.htm

Case Study #20: 52-Year-Old Joy Smith Given 6 Weeks To Live; Eliminates Stomach and Bowel Cancer Thanks To Cannabis

"According to the report published by The Daily Mail, Joy Smith was told she would only have six weeks to live when she was diagnosed with incurable stomach and bowel cancer in August 2016.

In a desperate attempt to defy expectations, she began taking a cannabis oil that contained THC, which is illegal in the United Kingdom (UK).

After a rollercoaster two years, she found out that she was cancer-free and would no longer have to have chemotherapy. Ms Smith, from Coventry, said: "I am going to party for the rest of my life. I have got to be the only person in the world who have survive this. I keep pinching myself to see if this is real. I am being monitored every three months, but other than that I have no more treatment planned."

Ms Smith was told that she would have little longer than a month left to live unless she started chemotherapy. Ms

Smith was unaware her friends had been researching an alternative cancer cure online until she was handed a cannabis-based tablet out of the blue. She admitted that she didn't want to take it at first because she 'didn't know what it was' – but did so anyway in the hope of a cure.

After taking regular doses of cannabis oil containing THC, her inoperable tumours almost completely disappeared. Ms Smith spoke about her battle against the cancer with the oil in March, when scans showed just a small amount of the disease left in her stomach. She was hopeful then that the cancer would completely disappear with continued cannabis oil use.

And Ms Smith said she hadn't stopped smiling since her appointment with her consultant on Monday, and said the news has yet to sink in. Ms Smith has received thousands of messages from fellow sufferers desperate to know more about her miracle cure, which has left doctors stunned.

Nearly two years on, doctors, who described Ms Smith as 'the luckiest woman in the world', are baffled as her scans show just a small amount of the disease is left in her stomach, which she is confident will disappear with continued cannabis use."

Source: https://guardian.ng/features/health/cannabis-oil-cures-stomach-cancer-as-new-genetic-diagnosis-identifies-men-six-times-more-likely-to-develop-prostate-tumour

Case Study #21: 74-Year-Old Man Cured of Bowel Cancer Thanks To Cannabis Oil

"I made the [cannabis] oil for my dad who is 74 and was diagnosed with bowel cancer at the end of July 2016. He had an operation to remove a large tumour from his bowel, and he still has at least three tumours in his liver.

He started chemotherapy in August and I made the oil for him and he started that at the same time. Mainly he's been taking big dollops at night - it's decarboxylated oil and super potent, but he enjoys the good night sleep and finally he's willing to administrate it himself, although he still has a few reservations about whether it can actually help - but sees no harm in giving it a go.

[He was undergoing] chemotherapy at the same time - which was making him feel terrible.

After three months of chemo he had his first scan – his tumours have shrunk by a third, and his blood cancer markers had gone down from 400 to 50, which is pretty amazing. **Every time he goes back for his chemo the doctors say how happy they are with his blood results.**

I've so far made oil out of three ounces of good quality Cannabis. I used the rice cooker method, after filtering the Cannabis using coffee filters, and then I decarboxylated it and left it in the oven for up to six hours. I then used around the same amount of coconut oil so it was less concentrated.

My dad has had big dollops at night (he's basically taken it every night since he started chemo) and I keep trying to get him to have more oil in the day through suppositories, which I think he'll finally start doing soon.

I don't know for a fact that the Oil is what's shrunk my dad's tumours so rapidly - but I have a feeling it's helping."

Source: www.cannabisoilsuccessstories.com/bowel-cancer-with-metastasis-to-the-liver.html

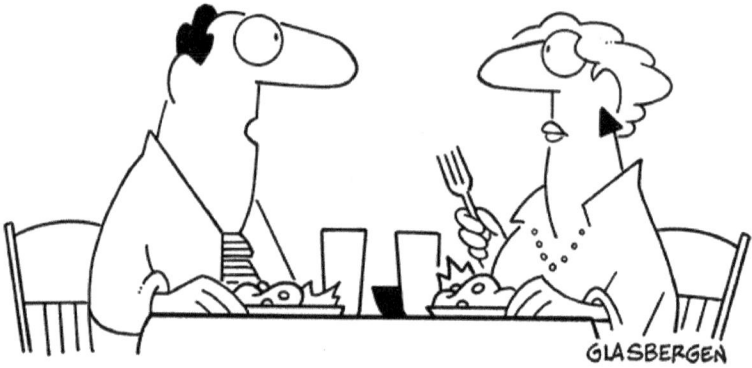

"On one hand, I'm troubled that one of my employees is using medical marijuana. On the other hand, it's nice that someone is actually laughing at my jokes."

Case Study #22: Hollywood Stuntman Mark Chavarria Claims Cannabis Oil Cured His Stage 4 Bowel Cancer

"Mark Chavarria saw his family doctor in September 2013, which led to a colonoscopy procedure in October. Unfortunately, the results of the test confirmed his biggest fear: Mark was diagnosed with stage four colorectal cancer. "I will beat this," he told his wife. "You watch me."

The tumours that had taken over Mark's body were enormous, consuming nearly 70 percent of his colon, as well as infiltrating his liver. The situation was dire.

One doctor told him the only solution was to surgically remove a portion of his colon and then fit him for a colostomy bag that he would have to wear for the rest of his life. Mark was mortified by the thought of such a drastic way out, especially since it make it impossible for him to continue a career as a Hollywood stuntman.

60

The next doctor suggested that while it might be possible for him to skip the colon-clipping surgery—at least for the time being—it was necessary to begin chemotherapy and radiation as soon as possible.

"I asked those guys if there was any way I could avoid surgery, and whether the chemo and radiation would get rid of the tumours 100 percent," Chavarria explained. "They said, 'nope, won't happen.'"

Without understanding what to really expect from this traditional cancer treatment, Mark launched full throttle into chemotherapy and radiation. The side effects were brutal, he explained. "I was in so much pain," he said. "I literally had to take Oxycontin and Hydrocodine just to go to the restroom.

Meanwhile, an old friend from high school **suggested that Mark try medical marijuana.** Mark was apprehensive because he believed that the concept of medical marijuana was just an excuse for stoners to get high. "I was raised that way," he said. "Drugs are bad."

By December, a caregiver in Colorado put Mark on a high-THC strain of cannabis oil, as well as provided him some raw herb to smoke. **"Once I got on this oil, I was able to get rid of everything,"** Mark explained, "all the Hydrocodine, the Oxycontin, everything."

The chemo and radiation caused Mark to lose a significant amount of weight—around 40 pounds within less than a year. Then something strange happened. In June of 2014, Mark woke up feeling different. "I just woke up and felt the cancer was gone from my body," he said.

Amazingly, at his next check-up, which included another colonoscopy and a CAT scan, **the doctor did not see any presence of tumours, only scar tissue from the**

radiation. Mark, who was about to learn he was cancer-free, screamed at the doctor, "Is it gone? Is it gone?"

Indeed, it was.

Throughout his battle with the deadly disease, Mark claimed he could tell the cannabis oil was attacking the cancer. "It's kind of gross, but I literally felt like I was pooping the thing out every time I went to the restroom," he explained. "What I believe happens with the oil is it makes like a shellac on the tumours, and it doesn't let it grow; doesn't let it breathe; doesn't let it eat... nothing. I think it was slowly, but surely, peeling away at the tumours like an onion."

Three of his friends, all roughly the same age, were diagnosed with stage four colorectal cancer around the same time. No matter how much Mark pleaded with them to give cannabis oil a try, they opted to listen to the doctors, who were always eager to experiment with the latest chemo and pharmaceutical drug. Sadly, all three perished under the advice and care of the American healthcare system. Mark, who is now living cancer-free and is back to work doing what he loves, believes that cannabis oil could have undoubtedly saved the lives of his friends. He urges anyone who has been diagnosed with cancer, even those living in states where marijuana is not legal, to find a way to get their hands on medical marijuana."

Source: https://hightimes.com/culture/hollywood-stuntman-claims-cannabis-oil-cured-his-stage-4-cancer

CHAPTER 6

Healing From Kidney Cancer

In this chapter, we look at the beneficial effects of cannabis extracts for kidney cancer.

Case Study #23: Cannabis Oil Reversed Linda Morado's Spreading Kidney Cancer

"In August 2014, Linda Morado received the most devastating news of her life – a diagnosis of Stage IV kidney cancer. It had metastasized to her lungs in two places. The month prior, Linda had also been diagnosed with celiac disease and nutrient malabsorption issues. Despite these overwhelming challenges, Linda was determined to live.

With eight years of experience in the United States Army, she intimately understands the value of a fighting spirit. She also has a large family to take care of, including five children, fifteen grandchildren, and two great grandchildren. Thankfully, through the power of cannabis extract medicine and unwavering spiritual belief, Linda is now cancer free.

Linda was given 10 months to live by her doctors. She underwent a surgery in an effort to extend her life, which included removal of her right adrenal gland and drainage of fluid in her right lung. After working through a number of emotions, Linda decided to use cannabis extract therapy.

The first oil she acquired was weak, which she discovered after four weeks of ineffectiveness led her to have a lab test conducted on it. It tested at 46% tetrahydrocannabinol (THC). The next batch was far stronger, testing at 85% THC. Within a couple months, Linda's energy and weight substantially improved, indicating the oil had positively impacted her condition.

A December 18, 2014 oncologist appointment revealed the lung cancer had disappeared, which surprised the doctor. He told Linda to continue doing what she was doing. **By January, the cancer was completely gone.**

She announced her recovery on a January 15, 2015 Facebook post: "I AM CANCER FREE!!! Stage 4 cancer and given a death sentence to cancer free in just a couple months!!!!! Hip Hip HORRAYYYYYYY."

A May 11, 2015, PET Scan confirmed Linda is still cancer free."

Source: https://illegallyhealed.com/linda-morado

Case Study #24: Simon Coleman's Recovery From Kidney Cancer Thanks To Cannabis Oil

"On 15th September 2012 I was diagnosed with a 4 inch tumour inside my right kidney. 99% confirmation of Renal Cell Carcinoma. The next week I discovered lots of information regarding cannabis and cancer. We Discovered the "Run from the Cure" documentary by

Rick Simpson. I continued researching and discovered a wealth of scientific evidence using cannabis oils. We soon discovered the dangers of radiation and chemotherapy. It soon became apparent, that it is usually the treatment that kills, more than the cancer itself. Still, at the advice of my doctor, on 15th October I had surgery to remove my right kidney.

On December 5th I received my pathology report. Aggressive renal Cell carcinoma with a sarcomatoid component. Grade 4 tumour (scale 1-4). The oncologist told us the cancer had burst out of my kidney into the surrounding fatty tissues and lymph nodes. I was stage 3 with a very bad prognosis.

I was offered and somewhat pressured into a clinical trial from a GSK sales rep and my oncologist, that offered zero guarantees of cure but certain devastating side effects ranging from Brain damage, liver damage, kidney damage and fatality, alongside many, many other organ complications. I'm 38 and otherwise very healthy. The treatment path they offer is total insanity in my opinion. You would be better off letting the disease takes its course rather than destroy your immune system and organs using their barbaric treatments.

On December 7th I started using Cannabis oil as my treatment choice. It is my human right to use any plant to save my life. The research shows non-toxicity with clear results of killing cancer cells in many, many cases. The evidence is out there. How any government can withhold and make illegal "A Plant" from anyone to cure their disease is a crime against humanity.

I have been using Cannabis oil (Rick Simpson oil) daily in what will be my life long battle against this disease. I follow the pH Miracle diet, keeping my system at a pH of 7.4. Cancer was discovered not to be able to survive in an alkaline system, many years ago.

65

[...] CT scan results January 5th 2013 came back, **I am Cancer free, no more cancer was detected in my lymph nodes.**

I have never felt healthier in my entire life. The cannabis oil, nutrition and diet changes have improved my health immensely."

[Note: see Simon's entire list of supplements and lifestyle changes at www.facebook.com/ricksimpsonofficial/posts/aggressive-renal-cell-carcinoma-with-a-sarcomatoid-component-grade-4-tumor-scale/490286517685159]

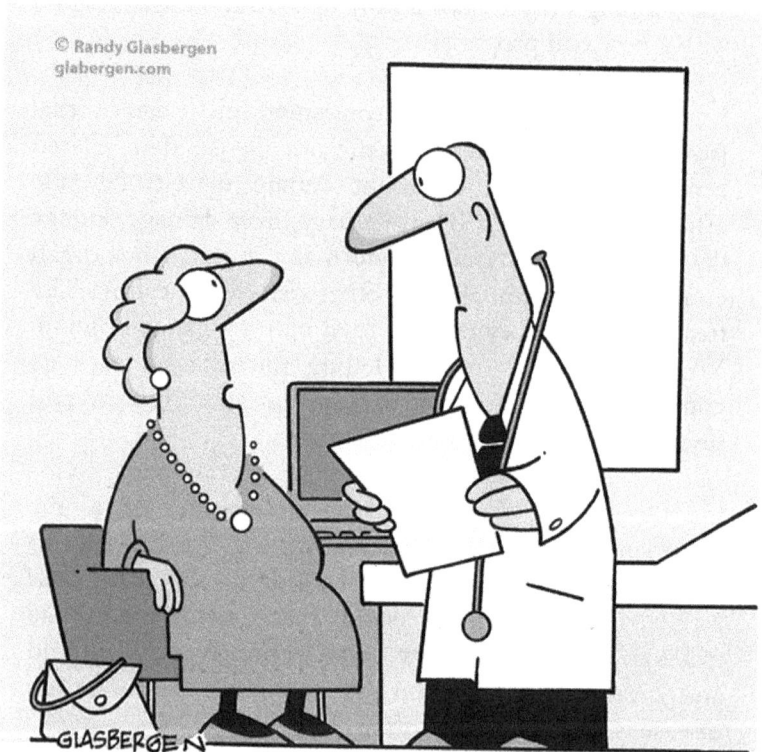

© Randy Glasbergen
glasbergen.com

GLASBERGEN

"Can you prescribe marijuana to help relieve the boredom of sitting in your waiting room?"

CHAPTER 7

Healing From Bladder Cancer

The following stories are about four remarkable individuals who decided to treat their bladder cancer naturally, with cannabis oil. The results they experienced speak for themselves.

Case Study #25: Trevor Smith Was Told He Had 2 Years To Live

"Trevor Smith, 54, a father-of-three, was diagnosed with bladder cancer in 2012. Doctors told him that without immediate surgery to remove his bladder, prostate and lymph nodes, followed by chemotherapy, he would be dead within two years.

Worried about his quality of life after such radical surgery, he decided to try alternative therapies and began taking cannabis oil after learning about it online.

Mr Smith, who works as a manager in the oil and gas industry, said, "It felt like I was going into the unknown, but the cannabis oil changed things for the better. When doctors told me I had gone into remission, I was lost for words, I almost couldn't believe it. I feel indebted to the oil and its properties. There are alternatives to chemo-therapy, but people just need to open their eyes to it."

Mr Smith's wife, Carol, 55, said, "So many thoughts rushed through my mind all at once when Trevor was diagnosed. All I could envisage was I was going to lose the love of my life. We knew we had to try a different approach to save his life."

While a healthy diet and alternative medicines, such as Essiac tea and vitamin supplements, were successful in improving Mr Smith's overall health, he was still in excruciating pain as the cancer continued to spread. It was then that they resorted to using cannabis oil to treat his cancer.

The couple from Derby made the controversial decision after discovering the documentary 'Run from the Cure', and arranged to pick up 60 grams of cannabinoid, an edible compound of the plant containing 65% tetrahydrocannabinol (THC). The couple, who have been married for 33 years, planned to carry out the treatment, which included feeding Mr Smith 60 grams of cannabis oil, over a period of ten weeks.

He claims that 10 weeks later, despite doctors' warnings about delaying treatment, the cancer had not spread to any other organs. He's now been cancer-free for a year."

Source: http://www.dailymail.co.uk/health/article-2725748/Cannabis-oil-helped-cured-cancer-claims-father-given-two-years-live.html

Case Study #26: Cannabis Extract Saved Her Life!

The carer of a 67-year-old woman from Colorado explains how cannabis oil cured her client's Bladder cancer and improved her quality of life:

"[Before cannabis extracts] She was in extremely poor health, her bladder cancer was addressed with chemo-therapy treatments every 6-9 month for the last six years, but the cancer kept returning. Chemotherapy had begun making her sick all the time and the doctor told her he would not be able to do chemotherapy anymore, so the next step was to remove the bladder.

For the COPD, she was on oxygen 24/7. She couldn't go more than a couple minutes without her oxygen. It was a constant battle keeping her out of the hospital with pneumonia. She had also had back injury over 20 years ago and was on morphine and muscle relaxers.

She was on morphine, extra-strength muscle relaxers, and a long list of pills; she had pills for everything.

[After using cannabis extracts] she got her life back; **just got her second clear report on the bladder cancer.** She no longer uses her oxygen and her O2 levels are around 93%. She has lost over 100 pounds! She no longer uses morphine or muscle relaxers.

She worked up to a gram of Cannabis Oil a day and continues to keep taking a daily gram each night. [The cannabis extracts] saved her life, no doubt!"

Source: www.cannabisoilsuccessstories.com/bladder-cancer-and-copd--67-yo-female.html

Case Study #27: 63 Year Old Man Given 3 Months To Live; Terminal Bladder Cancer Destroyed By Cannabis Oil

"I was given THREE months to live, with terminal cancer. I also had high blood pressure, diabetes, high cholesterol, and was overweight. I was a cripple, I couldn't walk, had no use of my upper girdle or arms. Vomiting 10 to 15 times a day. I broke four ribs from vomiting over 200 times.

[After taking cannabis oil] I have never felt this healthy in my life. **I am off all medications, fixed my diabetes, my blood pressure, my cholesterol.**

This gave me my life back. AND **I am cancer free.** I haven't even taken an aspirin, nothing, not one pill, since February 11, 2011.

I eat Cannabis in decarbed form. I ingest concentrated Cannabis Oil, I ingest coconut oil infused with Cannabis, and I vaporize.

Daily Cannabis intake:
- Three grams high-grade Cannabis Oil orally
- Two grams high-grade Cannabis Oil in suppositories
- One tablespoon of decarbed Cannabis in a smoothie
- Vaporized Cannabis flowers from 'good morning' until 'good night'
- Three to four Cannabis cookies
- 10ml of Cannabis-infused coconut oil

In six months I was off all my medications."

Source: www.cannabisoilsuccessstories.com/bladder-cancer--63-year-old-male---canada.html

Case Study #28: Bladder Cancer Free Using Cannabis Combined With Nutrition Protocol

"I was diagnosed with bladder cancer in June of 2016. I was completely surprised that I was 95% full of tumours.

I was told that the standard protocol for Bladder Cancer this aggressive was to immediately remove my bladder and be faced with wearing a bag or other options that I wasn't ready to accept. I immediately started researching alternative ways to deal with this other than surgery.

We found that a lack of nutrition was mostly to blame for cancers and we discovered that cannabis does indeed kill cancer cells and NOT healthy ones. **We also discovered that cancer is fed by sugar** and that a massive change in diet was in order if I wanted to become cancer free and stay that way!

One of the most important sites to read would be http://thetruthaboutcancer.com. Watch the video documentary series. It's very informative.

We next began taking Essiac Tea. If you've not heard about it, it's a Tea made from four different roots. It was passed on from an old Indian medicine man to a nurse in Canada named Rene Cassie.

In reference to nutrition I have found that the absolute best way to get massive organic whole foods into your body is through taking JuicePlus concentrated food capsules. Simply put it gives you incredible nutrition. I'll guarantee that 98% of people don't get their 8-13 servings of fruits and veggies a day! When you're fighting cancer you really need more than that.

I have been taking massive doses of Cannabis Oil in suppository form. By doing this you bypass the liver and you don't get high! The dose that I am taking is HUGE! It goes way beyond what you can buy at the local dispensary down the street here in Oregon. You could never be able to smoke or ingest as much as I do four times a day! I have mine specially made since the ones that we first started with weren't strong enough. The Cannabis definitely kills the cancer cells and not the healthy ones! I have had three surgeries now to clean out the tumours in my bladder. When I first started I was 95% full! **Now, seven months later, Nothing visible!**

I'll tell you now it's a whole lot easier fighting cancer with lots of love, support and prayers! I found that meditation and reading the word is also vital to healing. A positive attitude and NEVER SAYING "I have cancer" are very critical for me. I choose to say I am treating cancer SYMPTOMS! Not that I have cancer. I sincerely hope this can benefit someone."

Source: www.cannabisoilsuccessstories.com/t2a-bladder-cancer--59-yo-male.html

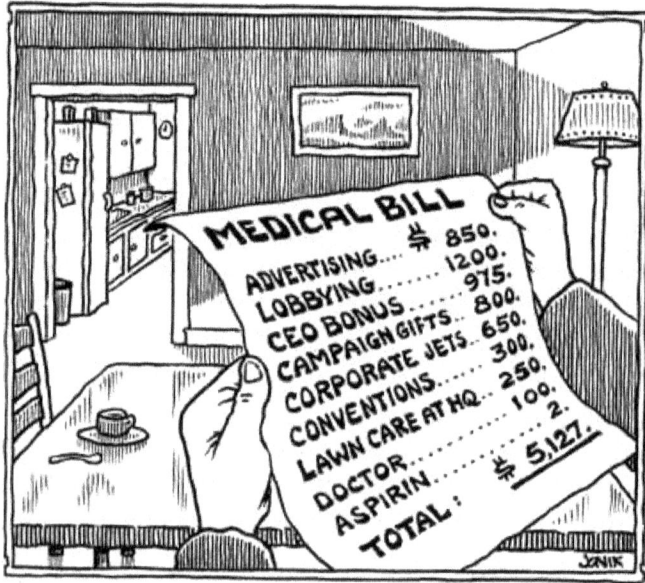

CHAPTER 8

Healing From Liver Cancer

Can cannabis oil help those suffering with liver cancer? The testimonials shared in this chapter will give you the answer.

Case Study #29: 100 Grams of Cannabis Extract in 90 Days to Treat Liver Cancer

"When dealing with cancer, it's always important to act quickly. Given the potential of tumours to grow or metastasize, early detection often is the key determinant of survival. John's experience exemplifies the importance of being proactive, no matter the diagnosis.

At the end of summer 2014, an ultrasound test showed the presence of two tumours in John's liver. Then, on September 3, 2014, John received the results of a CT scan which further analyzed the tumours, indicating one of them was already 2.5cm. While not confirmed, the tumours were thought to be hepatocellular carcinoma (HCC), a form of liver cancer; they could also have been high grade dysplastic nodules, which are pre-malignant tumours.

Between the ultrasound and CT tests, John and his wife Tracy researched alternative treatments and learned of cannabis oil. Due to their preparation, John was able to begin cannabis extract therapy the day he got his CT scan results.

John ingested 100 grams of full extract cannabis oil in 90 days. He ultimately ingested more than this, as he continued using a gram per day until mid-January. John never learned the cannabinoid profile of his oil but was assured it was regularly tested for quality and consistency.

John had to stop using cannabis oil in mid-January because he developed gallstones and became sick. Due to being in the hospital and trying to get that under control, he could not use any more cannabis oil until his next MRI. The results were received on March 7, 2015, which showed no more masses in John's liver. These results were surprising to John, his wife, and the oncologist.

Whether the tumours were actually HCC or had the potential to become HCC, it is never good to have tumours of any kind. John's quick actions ensured he did not even have the opportunity to find out.

In addition to using cannabis oil, John changed his diet and used turmeric, a widely consumed and healthful spice. John says combining cannabis oil with nutritional changes and other practices is important for optimizing the therapy's effectiveness."

Source: https://illegallyhealed.com/keep-calm-and-be-proactive

<u>Case Study #30: How Ed Moore Beat Stage IV Liver Cancer</u>

"My husband of 34 years was diagnosed with stage 4 primary liver cancer in March 2012. The doctor told us there was not much to be done since the tumour was 7 inches covering his lower lobe and also had spread to his lymph nodes.

We decided to go home and called hospice which gave us morphine for pain. Ed hated the morphine which made him vomit and also affected his mind. After one week at home we decided to do what we have done for many years, rely on ourselves. We choose a Naturopath doctor and have not had conventional treatments.

In our area we grow our own cannabis medicine and we started making Phoenix Tears (cannabis oil, 4 times daily, ½ gram each dose). Ed was off the morphine in one week after taking a gram of oil per day.

Later we added juicing fresh buds and leaves mixed with veggies. Ed is 65 and in excellent shape otherwise. Within a couple of weeks his pain and swollen stomach disappeared, and with it came hope.

He is also using a daily infrared sauna, epsom salt bath, and castor oil packs to get rid of toxins. We also do Vitamin C IVs with a Naturopath doctor.

We never saw an oncologist and only have done a blood test after the first diagnose CT scan. **His tumour marker went from over 6000 to normal and he is feeling well.**

He is up to 2 grams of phoenix tears now and does not feel stoned. I am also drinking the good tasting cannabis juice, with no effect. Not everyone could tolerate such a high dose of THC, but it works well for him."

"Supplements taken during the day include Green Tea, Multivitamin, Vitamin C, L-Proline / L-Lysine, Pancratin Enzyme, Liver Support Formula, Meriva-SR (Curcumin), Mushroom Immune Defense, Vitamin B17, Vitamin D, CoQ10, Selenium, Probiotics, Omega 3 Fish Oil, R-Lipoic Acid, N-Acetyl-L-Cysteine, Turmeric Extract, Milk Thistle, Papaya Leaf Extract. Ed also does castor oil packs and charcoal packs, alternating for several hours at night. These are great for getting the toxins out of his system.

Hospice just cancelled us, which is the first time they left a liver cancer patient go."

Source: www.chrisbeatcancer.com/ed-crushing-stage-four-liver-cancer-with-cannabis-oil

Case Study #31: Mike Cutler Was Sent Home With a Death Sentence

In 2009, Mike Cutler of the UK had a liver transplant. The procedure was an attempt to combat a bad case of liver cancer, but three years later, the cancer came back and attacked his new organ.

There was nothing his doctors could do. In his early 60s, Cutler was sent home from the hospital with ample amounts of morphine and a death sentence.

After being confined to bed rest and ill from morphine, Cutler knew there had to be another way. Armed with a laptop, he took to the internet, where he soon stumbled upon Rick Simpson's story.

He states: "Within three days, I'd stopped taking the morphine. My wife got me to go to the doctor's, and **he said "my God, you look well."** and he said "what's happening?" and I said, "well, I've stopped taking the morphine and I'm taking cannabis oil." And he was more concerned that I wasn't having serious withdrawal symptoms from stopping taking the morphine than he was about the cannabis oil.

About two months into taking the oil, I started coughing up blood. Or, what I thought was blood. And I thought, well this isn't good. My wife wasn't happy, so back to the doctor's we went. He took a sample and he looked at it, and he said "well, I don't know what this is, but it's not blood." It turns out, he was spitting out dead cancer cells.

When the results of Cutler's biopsy came back, he asked the doctors about his cancer. Their reply: "What cancer?"

After two months of cannabis oil treatment, Cutler's cancer couldn't be found."

Source: https://youtu.be/bxLkNLXUde4

Case Study #32: 58-Year-Old Masamitsu Yamamoto Saw a 95% Reduction In Tumour Markers Thanks To Cannabis

"After his 2010 diagnosis of Liver Cancer, Masamitsu Yamamoto underwent chemotherapy, but the cancer continued to spread. He then tried a wide variety of alternative therapies at great expense but without success. He says that in total, he has spent around ¥7 million trying to treat his cancer without success.

When he heard about medical marijuana being used as a cancer treatment, he made enquiries, but found there was no way he could obtain it legally in Japan. Since he did not want to support drug dealers, he began growing his own cannabis at home.

According to Yamamoto, using cannabis made him feel better and eased his depression, and his tumour markers fell to one twentieth of former levels (a 95% reduction)."

Source: www.japantimes.co.jp/news/2016/06/26/national/science-health/man-race-cancer-leads-japanese-fight-medical-use-marijuana

CHAPTER 9

Healing From Lymphoma

There are many stories and testimonials of people who have successfully treated their lymphoma using cannabis extracts. In this chapter, I share 4 of those remarkable stories.

Case Study #33: How Joanne Crowther Beat B-Cell Lymphoma

"This is Joanne Crowther's Story on how she beat Large B-cell lymphoma with Cannabis Oil.

In the summer of 2009 Joanne was diagnosed with large B-cell lymphoma. The lymphoma was eliminated with chemotherapy in February 2010. The treatment caused significant nausea, vomiting, febrile neutropenia (fever resulting from abnormally low white blood cell count), and pneumonia requiring hospitalization.

In March 2010, a brain MRI revealed several cancerous lesions. These were resolved by April 2010 with whole brain radiation, as indicated by a post-treatment MRI. For a year-and-a-half, Joanne was doing very well, even participating in a half-marathon. However, in November 2011, a mass developed in her left thigh. Doctors removed the 3.2 x 2.5cm mass, and determined it was consistent with large B-cell inter-vascular lymphoma.

The removal of this mass did not eliminate the lymphoma. In early January 2012, Joanne began receiving medications to treat complications of the cancer. Furthermore, another head CT scan revealed a 6mm cancer lesion in the left superior pons. The test also confirmed resolution of the previous lesions in the right thalamus and basal ganglia. Shortly after the 3.2 x 2.5cm mass excision, Joanne noticed regrowth of some mass in the same area. She received five shots of radiation in January for the new growth.

More scans in February 2012 revealed new adrenal cancerous nodules. Joanne began taking the chemotherapy drugs cisplatin and cytabarine to combat the cancers. She was then hospitalized between April 23rd, 2012 and May 3rd, 2012 due to acute renal failure and hepatitis, which had been induced by cisplatin and cytabarine respectively. The complications permanently ended Joanne's chemotherapy regiment in late April.

Joanne was then diagnosed with relapsed intravascular diffuse large B-cell lymphoma, and leptomeningeal disease. Without the strength to endure more chemotherapy or radiation, doctors could do nothing more, and **Joanne was forced to try an alternative treatment.**

In early May, she began taking cannabis oil. She started off with small rice-grain sized doses, but after a week felt no effects. She then upped her dosage to a gram of oil a day, and within two weeks noticed beneficial effects – in general, feeling better and having more appetite.

On July 30th, 2012, Joanne had a follow-up examination. It describes how Joanne is doing much better since being off chemotherapy, and that **the left thigh mass "actually regressed spontaneously."**

Two months later in another exam from September 24th, 2012 it states **Joanne is now in remission.** [...] Dr. John W. S. Yun stated, "She made a miraculous recovery with stable clinical condition."

Source: www.cureyourowncancer.org/joanne-crowthers-story-beating-large-b-cell-lymphoma-with-cannabis-oil.html

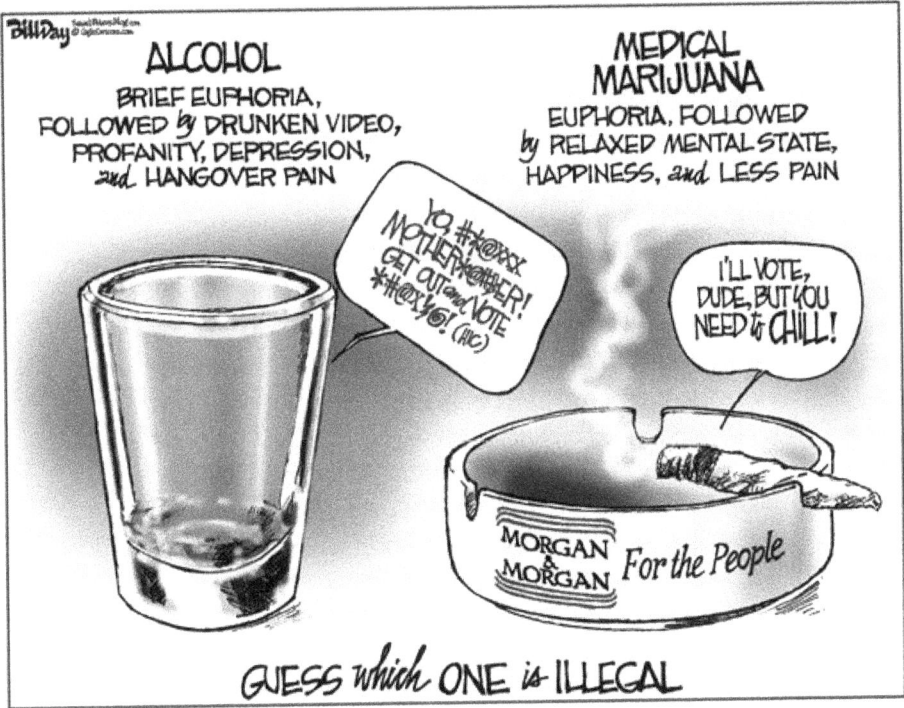

Case Study #34: Hodgkin's Lymphoma Cured with Cannabis Oil

"A while back, I read about Rick Simpson and cannabis oil and decided to try making some. I have been growing marijuana for a very long time. I used some of my best buds and made up some premium cannabis oil. I tried it and could not believe it. It was so potent it was like nothing I have ever had.

I knew of a patient that had been battling cancer (Hodgkin's Lymphoma) for about 11 years. I offered to be his medical marijuana caregiver and supply him with the oil at no cost to him so long as he would take the oil as recommended.

I had met him about a year prior at a compassion club meeting and learned then that he had the cancer. I really wanted to see if the oil could cure cancer, as mentioned in Rick Simpson's documentary 'Run from the Cure'.

After getting in contact with this patient and presenting the offer to him, we filed the proper paperwork with our state and began treatment. At first it was difficult for him because the oil was so potent and taking it three times per day can be quite difficult.

After three months, a very tumour on his upper chest started to shrink. After five months, the tumour was completely gone. He then went in for a CAT scan. The results came back that he is cancer free! The doctors have been trying to cure his cancer for at least 11 years. Chemo, bone marrow transplants, and so on. All it took was about a pound of premium bud converted into cannabis oil."

Source: www.cureyourowncancer.org/lymphoma-testimonials.html

Case Study #35: Tenille Farr Stopped The Spread Of Her Cancer In Its Tracks

"Tenille Farr is a devout Mormon. She grew up the fifth of nine children in small, rural, Rockland, Idaho. She served a mission for the Church of Jesus Christ of Latter-day Saints (LDS) before attending Brigham Young University, where she met her husband. They got married and she became the mother to five beautiful young boys.

While Farr was pregnant with her fifth son, Gabe, she was diagnosed with stage-2 Hodgkin's Lymphoma. If she underwent chemotherapy to treat the cancer, she risked losing Gabe or delivering him prematurely at severe risk to his health.

After much thought, prayer and research she decided to leave her family and home in Spanish Fork, Utah, to treat her cancer naturally with herbs and medical cannabis in Colorado and California, where the treatments are legal.

Through juicing whole-plant cannabis leaves and consuming full extract cannabis oil, she was able to stop the spread of her cancer, alleviate her symptoms and deliver a healthy baby this January.

Studies have shown there is no long-term risk to medical cannabis use in pregnancy. Research dating back to 1991 provides data on the development of 59 Jamaican children, from birth to age 5 years, whose mothers used marijuana during pregnancy.

Since returning home to Utah, Farr has stopped using cannabis. Her religious convictions, which are shared by 90% of the Utah state legislature, preclude her from breaking the law. She still has cancer that needs to be treated and some of her symptoms have returned.

You can follow Tenille on her blog, 'This Tale to Tell' a blog about courage and faith."

Source: https://illegallyhealed.com/treating-cancer-during-pregnancy

Case Study #36: Angela Harris, Diagnosed with Lymphoma, Outlives Her Prognosis By 20 Years

"Angela Harris never thought she would try cannabis, let alone suggest others use it. Harris is a conservative who grew up a devout member of the Church of Jesus Christ of Latter-day Saints (Mormon) in central California and Boise, Idaho. It wasn't until she saw the healing powers of cannabis that she tried it herself, and today she advocates and teaches others in conservative religious communities about plant medicines and alternative healing.

Angela says, 'I get that cannabis is a hard subject for families. The bottom line is that we have been lied to and we need to be able to be more open to that.'

Angela met her husband, Curt, a Utah native, at church in Boise. Curt and Angela have a lot in common: religion, humour and the desire to love and nurture an extended family. Angela was told when she was young that due to medical complications she would be unable to have children.

Now a mother of nine, Angela is a herbalist and medical cannabis advocate who has worked closely with legislators in her home state of Nevada as well as patients and legislators advocating for safe access in neighbouring Utah. She has made it her mission to advocate for change from within conservative communities like Utah, where cannabis is still highly stigmatized.

When Angela was pregnant with her sixth child, she was diagnosed with lymphoma. Because chemotherapy or other cancer treatments could cause potential harm to her unborn child and she had seen so many other people suffer using cancer drugs, she chose to treat her cancer naturally. Her only goal at the time was to deliver a healthy baby and die peacefully with her family.

Angela delivered a healthy baby girl, Abbigail, and went on to have three more children. She has outlived her prognosis by over 20 years. She and her family continue to research herbalism, or the use of plants as medicine, and have used the knowledge to help with friends and family who are suffering.

"The reason why cannabis is so important in Utah, and why this is such a key pivotal state, is because all other conservative state are looking at Utah to open the floodgates," she says. "It's time to talk about cannabis because too many people are suffering. Those of us who want a choice need a choice now."

Source: https://illegallyhealed.com/its-time-to-change-the-conservative-cannabis-conversation

The Power Of Your Mind

"A woman who had suffered constant poor health found, upon examining her beliefs, that she was telling herself: "Everyone gets sick," "There is so much disease around," "I catch everything," and "My body is fragile." Luckily, she was able to eventually turn her health around, by adopting new life-strengthening beliefs."

"We need to regularly reinforce our self-image in order to keep it healthy. We can do this by feeding our mind with positive, uplifting, inspiring thoughts about ourselves. [...] I repeated to myself over and over while in this meditative state, 'Every day in every way, I am getting better and better,' until I believed it. I imagined that the food I ate was 'energized,' making me healthier and healthier. Two months after I began reprogramming my mind, my doctor was amazed. He found no evidence of a tumour at all. He could not believe it. This is far from an isolated case. There are countless examples of health being restored using similar techniques. [...] Your body is a miraculous self-healing mechanism built to look after anything that happens to it. No doctor has ever healed a broken arm in his life. Only the body can heal the broken bones."

[...] "Nine-year-old Garrett Porter cured himself of a malignant tumour using a "Star Wars" visualization technique. It was estimated he had only about six months to live. Radiation treatments had failed. Surgery was out of the question. Using his mind he visualized his immune system as powerful. He visualized himself as the leader of a space fighter squadron fighting the tumour and winning, using the technique for twenty minutes each night. Five months later a brain scan was taken. The tumour was gone."

[...] "Athlete Kevin O'Neal saved his career by using the power of his mind. After a serious cycling accident, he visualized going inside his body and physically putting his broken bones together. The bones healed twice as fast as expected and he was able to compete."

John Kehoe, *Mind Power In The 21st Century*

CHAPTER 10

Healing From Prostate Cancer

Prostate cancer is the most common cancer in men and numbers are continually on the rise. In this chapter, you'll read testimonials of three men who have treated their prostate cancer whilst using cannabis.

Case Study #37: Cannabis Extracts Used To Treat Prostate Cancer

"Towards the end of my chemo, my oncologist was amazed at how healthy I was in spite of an intense chemo regimen that. I had plenty of side effects and am still healing from it all, but I had only lost about five pounds, have a good appetite, almost no nausea, lost my beard, but not all my hair, feet and fingers were sore, but not raw, and developed no mouth or throat lesions.

She wanted to know how this could be and I told her that I wasn't taking any of the other medicine prescribed, but just ingesting Cannabis Oil during the worst days of my chemo side effects.

The Cannabis Oil was made by a family member using 190 Everclear and flower tops. I took the oil and made my suppositories as best I could with organic coconut oil.

Suppositories were half of a gram twice a day. Worked full time in a zero-tolerance environment until I started chemo and I was delighted that there was no high with the suppositories. For the chemo side effects, I built myself up to ingesting half of a gram a day, twice a day, and might even have eaten a little more on the real bad days. I stopped the suppositories because of diarrhoea induced by the chemo.

There is no way I will ever know for certainty that it was the Cannabis that produced such unexpected results, but what else could it be? **My PSA dropped after the initial post-surgery test and the PSA out to Mayo. That, too, was unprecedented.** And the only deviation from the standard treatment was the Cannabis."

Source: www.cannabisoilsuccessstories.com/prostate-cancer--advanced.htm

Case Study #38: Dennis Hills' Prostate Cancer Eliminated In 3 Months with Cannabis Oil

"Three years ago, after a prostate biopsy, I was given the diagnosis of aggressive Stage III adenocarcinoma. I didn't know what to do. The urologist made appointments for me to start radiation, and maybe chemo. Then a friend told me cannabis cures cancer. It just so happened that the first human trials of cannabis treatment of astrocytomas (inoperable brain cancer), were published with encouraging results. So, I decided rather than die from the medical treatment, I would do the cannabis cure.

There was no dispensary in the area, but a friend made me cannabis butter, so I took that up to tolerance. **In three months, the primary cancer was gone,** only minor metastatic lesions were left. At that point I found a supplier for Rick Simpson's oil **and killed off the metastases in the next three months.** Now I just take a maintenance dose of locally produced hash oil that is 1:1 THC:CBD with about a 30% potency. This will certainly keep me clear of cancer, anywhere, forever.

My point in telling this story is the fact that in the face of advanced aggressive cancer, all I had was very weak cannabutter, but it was enough to eliminate the primary tumour. Now there are strains of 95% THC. But is this necessary? If you have cancer and want to pursue the cannabis treatment, any at all will be good. More important than extreme potency is balance between THC and CBD. If you can get high potency, great. If not, common potencies will work perfectly."

The well-known anxiolytic property of cannabis provides an improvement in quality of life in all facets of living in the world. It is so sublime to feel contented well-being going through this process of healing. Sure beats life in a hospital."

Source: www.cureyourowncancer.org/dennis-hills-story-beating-prostate-cancer-with-cannabis-oil.html

Case Study #39: Paul Morrissey Says Cannabis Oil Is Beating His Prostate Cancer

A St. John's man suffering from prostate cancer that had metastasized is crediting marijuana oil treatment with putting him on the mend.

"It makes me feel 20 years younger, that's what the marijuana oil does," said Paul Morrissey, adding he shovelled snow for three hours during the recent blizzard and blackout with no problems.

"There was pretty ferocious wind and snow. I came out of it looking like a walking popsicle. However after all that work and so forth I was in excellent condition. Even without cancer, I wouldn't suspect I'd last that long or do that well."

Morrissey's prostate-specific antigen (PSA) blood levels have improved dramatically and there has been some regression in his lymph nodes and abdomen.

Morrissey's PSA levels dropped nearly 10 times from their previous level — down to 3.3 from 29.5.

Morrissey said he did take pill medication for roughly a month and an injection prescribed by his oncologist, but is so convinced the oil was what helped him, he has discontinued the course of conventional treatment. He hasn't received any chemotherapy or radiation either.

The Telegram first told Morrissey's story in September 2013 when he said at Stage 4 prostate cancer, he was putting his faith in the cannabis oil treatment. Morrissey insists his PSA levels plummeted because of six weeks on the cannabis oil.

He was sold on the controversial treatment after watching a documentary by Rick Simpson, called "Run from the Cure." Morrissey said that on his way to Toronto in December 2012, he spent five hours with Simpson. "Four people in that house had cancer," Morrissey said last fall. "They cured themselves."

Source: www.cureyourowncancer.org/cannabis-oil-is-beating-prostate-cancer-paul-morrisseys-story.html

CHAPTER 11

Healing From Brain Cancer and Brain Tumours

In this chapter, I share with you eight stories of incredible people who chose to go against the mainstream and treat their brain cancer and tumours using cannabis oil. The results are truly remarkable.

Case Study #40: Kristen Okimura's Natural Approach to Aggressive Brain Cancer

"Glioblastoma multiforme (GBM) is one of the most aggressive and fatal brain cancers in existence. Most patients die within two years of diagnosis. However, an increasing number of patients are turning to cannabis oil as a potential treatment for many brain cancers, given the promising anecdotal and scientific evidence.

Kristen Okimura's experience is a testament to how important and effective cannabis extracts really can be.

Kristen had a seizure on April 7, 2014, which led to a hospital stay. Within days she was diagnosed with GBM and had surgery to remove the tumour. Without understanding the impact of this decision, she also had a chemotherapy wafer inserted, which releases relatively small amounts of chemotherapeutic agents and dissolves in 2 to 3 weeks. This chemo wafer exempted her from participating in many clinical trials.

Since surgery cannot remove all cancerous cells, doctors recommended chemotherapy and radiation to prevent recurrence. **Without these additional treatments Kristen was given four and a half months to live.**

Due to her mom's experience with breast cancer, in which years of radiation and chemotherapy failed to permanently eradicate the disease, Kristen decided to take a natural approach.

A doctor relative of Kristen's introduced her to the potential of cannabis oil to directly fight her cancer. With the support of her husband, Kristen took immediate action and was using cannabis oil within three weeks of diagnosis. Her professional background in environmental testing instilled in her a deep respect for the importance of data and consistent tracking of results.

She put together a schedule and monitored her daily responses to cannabis oil doses over several months. By doing this, Kristen was able to create a dosing regimen and routine.

Kristen used two different kinds of full extract cannabis oil when fighting her cancer. The first was an extract with a 1:1 ratio of THC:CBD. She also had a high-THC oil, which was especially hard to tolerate. Therefore, Kristen developed a schedule where she consumed the 1:1 oil at 10:00am, 2:00pm, and 6:00pm, and then the high-THC oil at 10:00pm. These doses totalled to 0.9 grams per day.

As a mother of two children, Kristen sometimes deviated slightly from this schedule due to parenting responsibilities, but for the most part she has been able to strictly adhere to it.

She has had stable MRIs since the tumour was removed, and **her oncologist is continually amazed with Kristen's continued success with the cannabis oil protocol.**

In addition to using cannabis oil, Kristen mastered her nutrition and exercised daily. She already had good habits before the diagnosis, so continuing to live well was not hard for her. Kristen believes that the combination of nutrition and cannabis oil is likely why the cancer has not returned."

Source: https://illegallyhealed.com/kristens-natural-treatment-plan-for-aggressive-brain-cancer

Case Study #41: Lynn Cameron Was Given 6-18 Months To Live – She Is Alive And Well 4 Years Later

"No one wants to be told they have cancer — let alone an inoperable brain tumour, yet this is the exact reality Lynn Cameron was faced with in 2013.

In December of that year, doctors informed the 48-year-old that she had just "six to 18 months" to live. You can imagine her devastation. Determined to live, Cameron underwent several sessions of chemotherapy along with radiotherapy.

"I had a seizure on November 30, 2013, prior to which I had been quite well. I had a scan on December 10 and it showed a mass, and I was taken straight into Glasgow's Southern General at that point," explained Cameron. "I was operated on December 16, and on December 27 **I was told that I had stage 4 terminal brain cancer.** So I underwent the chemotherapy and radiotherapy, but was told even then I would live six to 18 months at best."

Scared by the diagnosis, she also began supplementing with cannabis oil (CBD) — a therapy that is presently illegal in the UK. **"A good friend suggested cannabis, but I was too scared because it's illegal.** I also found it hard to believe that it would cure brain cancer so advanced," she said. "But as the scans were showing there was no change to the mass, I eventually thought, 'I'm going to break the mould here and try that'."

Nearly four years after her diagnosis, Lynn is still alive and says cannabis oil is the reason. She is now advocating "for the reform of the current prohibitive laws around the use of cannabis for medication."

Over the past four years, the cancer patient has educated herself on a wide range of natural therapies to combat the affliction. She said, "I researched more and more into natural 'cancer killers' and decided to follow an alkaline diet and cut out processed foods altogether. I also cut out sugar completely. I started taking cannabis oil under my tongue, as it gets straight into the blood stream that way."

Reportedly, every scan Cameron received showed an improvement. **"By the sixth MRI, the cancer had gone,"** she said.

"Doctors had told me, 'eat whatever you like, take all the vitamins you want, it won't work'. **But these were the people who told me my cancer was incurable, and yet it was gone,"** she exclaimed.

Source: www.naturalnews.com/2017-09-12-cancer-survivor-says-cbd-oil-saved-her-life-after-doctors-said-she-had-6-months-to-live.html

Case Study #42: 45-Year-Old Man Paralyzed By Cancer, Now Able To Walk Thanks To Cannabis

"A 45-year-old male who lives in the U.K. was diagnosed with Brain cancer. He was given two to four weeks to live, and all treatment was stopped by doctors. He was paralyzed down his right-hand side and unable to speak or walk moved to a Hospice.

Initially, he was given Chemotherapy, radiotherapy, steroids, as well as medication to stop his fits. As a final effort to save his life, he turned to cannabis extracts. Now, he is able to talk clearly, move his right-hand side, and walk a short distance.

He took 0.5 mil 50/50 THC rectally, because oral dosing made him too high. Two mil CBD 30% full spectrum orally, and he also vapes CBD as needed.

His brother has this to say: 'I feel if we had believed what the doctors had said and not found out about Cannabis Oil, my brother would have died. **I truly believe it has helped my brother and cannot believe you are banned from using it in the UK.** Cannabis Oil needs to be tried by the hospital as a cure for cancer. He has now moved out of the hospice and gone home.'"

Source: www.cannabisoilsuccessstories.com/brain-cancer--45-yo-male.html

Case Study #43: Brain Tumour Vanishes In 'Miracle Baby' After Family Chooses Cannabinoid Oil

"There is nothing quite so horrendous and heartbreaking as a baby with a malignant brain tumour, especially for parents and family. But at the same time, there is little as joyous and uplifting as seeing those tumours go away – and without the costly "assistance" of the corporate medical industry.

Recently, the father of an eight-month-old baby decided he would shun traditional radiation treatment and chemotherapy and instead push for an alternative treatment using cannabis oil. The baby's physician, Dr. William Courtney, who was initially sceptical earlier in his career about medical cannabis, has since seen such impressive results with it that he's now a big believer and a staunch advocate.

"They were putting cannabinoid oil on the baby's pacifier twice a day, increasing the dose... And within two months there was a dramatic reduction," Courtney said in an interview with *The Huffington Post*.

At four months the tumour had completely disappeared, and after eight months of treatment, the brain architecture and tissues were completely normal.

The physician further noted that successful application of cannabis in this case means that "this child is not going to have the long-term side effects that would come from a very high dose of chemotherapy or radiation... currently the child's being called a miracle baby, and I would have to agree that this is the perfect response that we should be insisting is frontline therapy for all children before they launch off on all medications that have horrific long term side effects."

[...] [Studies show that] benign tumours in other organs, such as the pancreas, testes, uterus and mammary and pituitary glands, were diminished as well. Several reviews also found that cannabinoids appear to encourage cancer cell death (apoptosis), while preserving normal cells. Moreover, cannabis induces programmed cell death in breast cancer cell lines and offers protection against both colorectal and lung cancer.

CNN's chief medical correspondent, Dr. Sanjay Gupta, says it's time for a "medical marijuana revolution."

Source:www.naturalnews.com/056022_cannabis_oil_brain_tumours_medical_marijuana.html

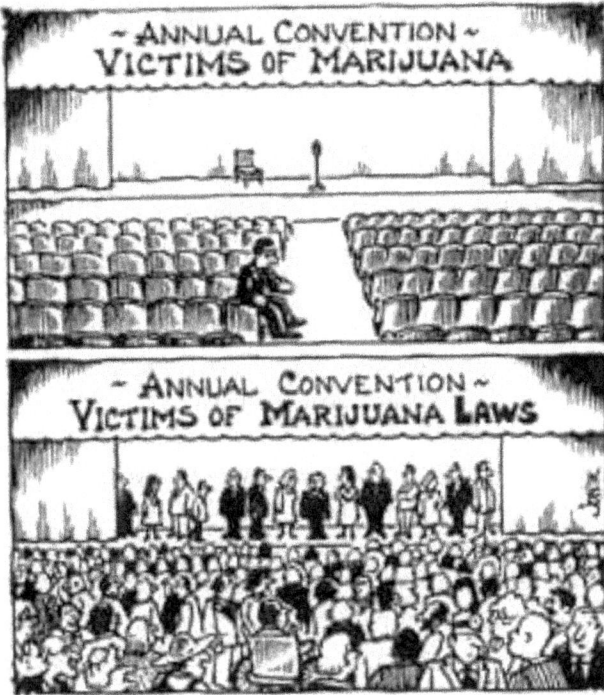

Case Study #44: Diagnosed With Glioblastoma and Given 3 Months To Live... Saved Thanks To Cannabis Extracts

"On March 3, 2009 I had emergency brain surgery ten days after the birth of my fourth child. They removed a tumour which I wasn't expected to live from. The surgery left me extremely epileptic and the medications I was given did not control the seizures. The medications also let me with extreme physical side effects. I lost two pregnancies due to epilepsy medication.

In 2014 **I was diagnosed with an intrinsic brainstem glioma and given three months to live.** I performed a complete lifestyle and diet change and increased my use of Cannabis Oil; the tumour stopped growing. In 2015, I quit all pharmaceutical medications with the exception of potassium, which is a form of salt.

On March 9, 2016 I gave birth to my fifth child. Her entire pregnancy was supported by the consumption of oral medical cannabis oil in large quantities. This was monitored by the University of Washington hospital. **Ahyoka would never had been born, nor would I be alive, without the use of medical Cannabis Oil.**

The Oil is the only medication I have been able to find that controls my epilepsy enough to function normally. Ahyoka is incredibly healthy, very smart, and has no negative side effects due to my Cannabis use. **The last time I had an MRI in December 2016 they did not see any brain tumours.** Cannabis oil saved my own and my daughter's lives."

Source: www.cannabisoilsuccessstories.com/glioblastoma--40-yo-female.html

Case Study #45: Oligodendroglioma Brain Tumour: Choosing Cannabis Over Chemo

"I took Full Extract Cannabis Oil (FECO), either bought from a dispensary or homemade. I either dispensed it on a cracker or dispensed it into empty gel caps. I took a high THC, usually around 55%, with practically no CBD (usually less than 1%). I took a hybrid and sativa depending on what was available at the dispensary. I supplemented with a CBD tincture, and other CBD products. I took up to six CBD (Harlequin and AC/DC) flower bud packed gel caps a day in addition to the oil. These had not been decarboxylated. I also used a vape pen with various oils.

My goal was the Rick Simpson protocol: 60 grams of Cannabis Oil within 90 days. I started with a dose half the size of a grain of rice and tried to double it as often as I could until I achieved one gram a day.

I spread the dose out equally throughout the day, sometimes taking as much as ten caps a day. I did this protocol twice, with five weeks in-between where I was just on a maintenance dose of 0.10 grams of FECO.

The last two weeks of the second protocol, I was taking two grams a day. I used a high THC Cannabis Oil, (usually around 55%) and low CBD (usually less than 1%) in a hybrid and/or sativa and sometimes I could find an Indica. I also took up to six or so caps spread throughout the day of non-decarboxylated CBD buds (Harlequin and AC/DC) packed into a gel cap.

I also took a CBD tincture spray at nightly before bed and I vaped CBD and THC oil during the day as often I could.

I am beyond grateful that I chose Cannabis Oil over chemo! My gut feeling was to refuse chemotherapy and look for alternatives. I am now living a dream life in the Sierra Nevada mountains of California; hiking and enjoying every blessed day!"

Source: www.cannabisoilsuccessstories.com/oligodendroglioma-brain-tumour.html

Case Study #46: Sophie's Story: Healing an Optic Pathway Glioma Brain Tumour

"There were no treatments before cannabis. Three months prior to the beginning of Sophie's chemotherapy treatment, she began cannabinoid therapy.

The only side effects she ever had was a little sleepiness that completely went away as she acclimated to the oils, and hunger, which is amazing since the chemotherapy can affect her appetite. Some of the miracles Sophie has experienced on Cannabis Oil are as follows:

- Perfect Vision! Doctors said Sophie would have partial if not complete blindness with zero chance of saving her vision. Due to the shrinkage we have seen from the use of Cannabis Oil, they have saved her vision, which after an eye exam was reported to be "that of a normal child"
- After nine blood transfusions, Sophie stopped needing them one day while still on chemotherapy, which is considered medically impossible
- She's only been neutropenic once, and doctors believe that was due to a cold
- **Total tumour shrinkage for 19 months, despite her doctor saying the best-case scenario would be 4-6 months**
- Despite over two-and-a-half years of chemotherapy, Sophie has continued to gain weight and has had a great quality of life, has a full head of hair and she is advancing developmentally."

Sophie has been on lab tested (free of pesticide, mould, residual solvents and microbiologicals) high THC and CBD concentrated Cannabis Oils infused with MCT or "fractionated coconut oil" with a recent addition of THCa in an organic olive oil tincture over the last 12 months. Her first year, she used ethanol oil, and in the two years since, she has used CO2 oil that includes terpene reintroduction. As for strains: THC strains - Isabella's Bloom (CannaKids Proprietary strain), Girl Scout Cookies, Blue Dream, Cotton Candy Diesel, Purple OG. CBD strains - AC/DC, Cannatonic, Ringo's Gift, Valentine X.

Her initial target dose was 450mg at a ratio of 2:1, THC:CBD. We then changed it to a 1:1 ratio and saw very little differences in the amount of shrinkage that occurred. We then changed it to a 3:1 ratio, CBD:THC at 400mg of total active cannabinoids per day, and also layered in 50 mg of THCa into the regimen – this was adjusted this way to try to stop any potential tumour growth that would be a direct result of her hitting intense growth spurts, which in turn feed the tumour.

Hands down, Cannabis Oil has saved my daughter in more ways than I could ever imagine or explain! Putting her on Cannabis Oil at such a young age, prior to starting chemotherapy, was the best decision our family ever made."

Source: www.cannabisoilsuccessstories.com/optic-pathway-glioma-brain-tumour-and-cannabis-oil-success.html

Case Study #47: Anaplastic Astrocytoma: Taking A Chance On An Alternative Method

A 54-year-old female from Colorado successfully treated her Grade 3 Anaplastic Astrocytoma with cannabis oil.

"The original diagnosis was a grade 2 astrocytoma in 2005. I did oral chemotherapy, no radiation. Three tumours recurred in 2015, two of which were in the resected cavity. One was inoperable, located in the thalamus area.

I took Keppra for seizures for a couple of months but didn't like the side effects so I stopped that, and started taking CBD oil as suggested by my Neuro-Oncologist at UCSF.

I started taking Cannabis Oil in June of 2016. By November the tumour in the thalamus was gone, the other tumours were stable. I continued using Cannabis Oil, and my last MRI in February showed 'no evidence of disease'.

I used a 1:1 ratio Cannabis Oil, strains unknown, once a day before bed. I take an amount of Cannabis Oil about the size of a lentil bean.

I was never a recreational user. **I was totally against it, but when I got cancer I did my research and decided to take a chance on the alternative method. I'm sure glad I did.**"

Source: www.cannabisoilsuccessstories.com/anaplastic-astrocytoma-grade-3--54-yo-female.html

CHAPTER 12

Healing From Leukaemia

Before sharing with you three case studies relating to the effect of cannabis on Leukaemia, I would like to preface this chapter by quoting an article that appeared in 2017 in www.NaturalNews.com, titled *"Cannabis Phytochemicals Found to be Effective in Destroying Leukaemia Cells"*:

> "Researchers from St. George's, University of London have confirmed that cannabinoids are effective in destroying the cells of leukaemia, a cancer of blood-forming organs. When used in conjunction with chemotherapy treatments, cannabinoids, the active chemicals in cannabis, results against the blood cancer cells improved significantly. The new findings, which have been published in the *International Journal of Oncology*, suggest that lower doses of chemotherapy can be administered to patients."

Case Study #48: Three-Year-Old Boy with Leukaemia Given Days to Live

"In another of the many stories that have emerged of cancer being successfully treated with cannabis oil, **a three-year-old boy in Utah who was given just days**

to live by doctors because of leukaemia is thriving thanks to the oil. After two months of chemo, Landon Riddle was refusing to eat and vomiting dozens of times a day. After researching cannabis oil treatment online, his family travelled to Colorado to gain access to it. After just a few days, his vomiting eased, his appetite returned, and he was showing signs of improvement. **Months after the ordeal, he, too, was free of cancer.**

The family, fed up with the fact that the only treatment doctors could recommend was chemotherapy – even after little Landon Riddle kept vomiting dozens of times daily and refused to eat after two months of chemo – looked into cannabis oil treatment. They travelled to Colorado where such a treatment is legal.

"His whole chest was full of leukaemia tumours which is why he couldn't breathe," says his mother, Sierra. "They started him on chemo but told us that he probably wasn't going to make it. We discussed all of our concerns with his medical team in Utah and watched Landon continue to suffer and wither away as they piled on drug after drug." But rather than give in to a death sentence and play into Big Pharma's only recommendation, Landon began cannabis oil treatments. The results have been incredible.

Within just days of the treatment, Landon showed signs of improvement. Instead of withering away, his appetite surged, and his vomiting lessened. He rebounded, and as explained on a CNN video, **is still cancer-free even months later."**

Source:www.naturalnews.com/051881_cannabis_oil_cancer_treatment_Big _Pharma.html

Case Study #49: Hairy Cell Leukaemia Treated Successfully with Cannabis Within 6 Months

"[Before I took Cannabis] I was tired or exhausted mentally with bad brain fog, profuse bleeding from pinpricks, I felt angry, overwhelmed by everything, and had a headache 24/7. I slept 12 hours at night and took a two to three-hour nap in the late afternoon.

[After I started taking Cannabis] my energy returned, brain fog is gone, I'm getting eight hours of sleep with a much shorter nap in the late afternoon (not uncommon before the illness), bleeding time is markedly shorter as scabs form quickly, and there are no headaches. I'm much more content and peaceful, feel ease in living life and I'm dealing with activities of daily living.

We grew our own cannabis, about five different strains including both indica and sativa strains. Tested out at about 60% THC. I recall strains such as Jack Herer, White Widow, ABC, and some others whose names escape me. We also used the Gerson Therapy for an anti-cancer diet and lifestyle. We added turmeric milk the last six months and are continuing permanently.

[Dosing]: I took about a half gram a day for two years. The first 18 months, we bought at dispensaries, but my condition was only stable and slightly improved when our crop matured, and we made our own. **Within 6 months (of using our home-grown medicine) my blood was essentially normal** with only the platelets low, but no longer dangerously so. I take a maintenance dose at night.

Because the diagnosis was for an incurable form of cancer, we were amply warned that the chemo-cladribine-would fail within ten years, leaving the leukaemia harder to treat, requiring another round of more cladribine in larger doses and probably another adjunct called ritaximbab (that's not the correct spelling) which prior medical victims reported as extremely unpleasant.

This made our decision to forego their recommend-dations very easy! I'm a Cannabis enthusiast but did not enjoy the psychological effects of Cannabis Oil and therefore took less than the recommended dose, however, it worked eventually anyway. **I have my life back, feel good again, and I'm enjoying life like a normal person.** We no longer fear this disease because we know what to do now."

Source: www.cannabisoilsuccessstories.com/hairy-cell-leukemia.htm

Case Study #50: Nine Year Old Mykayla Heals From Leukaemia

Nine year old cancer patient Mykayla was diagnosed with T-cell Acute Lymphoblastic Leukaemia (a cancer of the blood and bone marrow). This is a very rare and aggressive form of childhood leukaemia; it accounts for 15-18% of childhood leukaemia cases.

She was headed toward full body radiation and a bone marrow transplant, but her parents refused to let her endure this suffering and instead opted to use cannabis oil. After six days of use, Mykayla was in remission.

Her parents write: "Mykayla's DNA was altered somehow and it caused her bone marrow to start producing immature/leukemic white blood cells. These immature white blood cells are known as "lymphoblasts".

Mykayla fell ill in May of 2012. She had flu like symptoms such as body aches, fevers, fatigue, cough, and runny nose. She was evaluated by an urgent care office and diagnosed with strep throat. They prescribed antibiotics but she did not get better. She soon developed a red rash on her ankles.

Her bruises that covered her body were alarming to us… as she was too tired to play outside where she normally got bruises like this. Her tummy began to hurt badly and we took her to her paediatrician. He wanted us to remove dairy from her diet, to see if that solved the issues we were having, but it continued to get worse.

She began sweating during the night, so badly that it would soak through her sheets into her mattress. Her breath was shallow… and her skin was pale, and cool to the touch. Her heart beat was funny, but we couldn't pin-point what exactly was different. We feared that we would lose her if they did not find out what was wrong.

On Friday, July 13th 2012 we took Mykayla back to the paediatrician. While checking for pneumonia they discovered a basketball sized mass (of lymphoblasts) in her chest. We were sent to Portland Oregon where the nearest children's hospital is and the very next day she underwent spinal taps and bone marrow biopsies and was subsequently diagnosed with Leukaemia.

Mykayla's mass was so large that she was not able to be sedated for risk of death from the pressure on her oesophagus and heart. Some of the valves that drain fluid from around her heart were blocked by the mass causing her pericardial effusion (fluid around the heart). She spent 3 days in the Intensive care unit and had to undergo an entire surgery to place a PICC line with no anaesthetic or pain relief at all due to the risk it posed on her condition.

Her Treatment

In the United States of America there are only TWO approved treatments for cancer… radiation and chemotherapy. Both are extremely toxic to the human body. When you are a child with cancer your parents do not have the option to refuse the approved way without facing legal repercussions that could include losing custody of the child. [...] Our family strives to provide Mykayla with the best possible chance of living a normal and healthy long life. With these thoughts in mind I will explain Mykayla's treatment in further detail.

We have chosen the very basic chemotherapy protocol for childhood leukaemia available to satisfy the "approved" and required treatment.

We had a plan from the very beginning to combat Mykayla's cancer naturally and **that was to use cannabis in the form of very concentrated and potent oil, raw cannabis juice, and cannabis cooked into food.** Cannabis has been known to kill cancer, protect the body from the damage of chemotherapy, relieve pain and nausea, and it is a neuroprotectant and antioxidant.

Mykayla began cannabis therapy on July 24th 2012! Instantly she was able to eat again. That was the first benefit that we noticed. She was happier, she smiled and laughed constantly. We loved it! One week after we began the oil treatment Mykayla's physicians notified us that her leukaemia had vanished from her bone marrow and blood! She was in remission. Never again will I fear cancer... We found the answer!

Besides 'Cannabis oil', this medicine has many names: Full Extract Cannabis oil (FECO), Rick Simpson Oil (RSO), Whole Plant Extract are the most common...

All strains possess their own benefits, they are all beneficial... Blending strains gives you a broad spectrum cannabis oil with a wide variety of positive benefits... When You are treating cancer with cannabis oil, you need all cannabinoids, not just THC or CBD...

July 14th 2012 (diagnosis day and steroid treatment began) Mykayla's Lymphoblast percentage in her blood smear was 33% July 15th 2012 – 51% July 16th 2012 – 11% (began chemotherapy) July 17th 2012 – 14% July 18th 2012 – 16%

July 19th 2012 – 3% July 20th 2012 – 29% (got released from hospital) July 23rd 2012 – 31% July 24th 2012 – **BEGAN CANNABIS OIL** July 26th 2012 – **5%.** July 30, 2012 - **3%** blasts August 2nd 2012 – **0%** blasts August 6th 2012 – **0%** blasts August 13th 2012 – **0%** blasts August 20th 2012 – **0%** blasts TODAY – **0%** blasts!

July 30th 2012 was THE VERY LAST TIME THEY HAVE FOUND LYMPHOBLASTS IN MYKAYLA'S BLOOD SMEAR!!!! **The very next time we saw the oncologist they told us Mykayla was in remission.**

Some may say that cannabis does not "cure" cancer… but this right here shows something… proof enough for me! Some say cannabis is inappropriate for children… We say cancer is inappropriate for children.

Diet is medicine. Cancer thrives in an acidic environment and is fed by sugar. We try our best to create a diet for Mykayla that is healthy, vegetarian (vegan if she will tolerate), organic, with no artificial additives, preservatives, or dyes. We also give her tons of alkali water.

Supplements work wonders. Some important supplements that we have found helpful in the fight against cancer and chemotherapy are. Vitamin C, Green Tea extract, Milk Thistle, Beta Carotene, coconut oil, vitamin D, essiac tea, COQ10, selenium, omega 3, garlic, cannabis, and tons of fruits and vegetables.

Having a positive attitude and providing your child with a happy, bright, and loving home provides a better outside environment to fight cancer in. I believe strongly that the love and happiness that our family values dearly has to do with the success that we have seen Mykayla have while battling leukaemia."

Source: www.bravemykayla.com/her-treatment.html

CHAPTER 13

Other Types of Cancer

In this chapter, you'll discover how cannabis extracts can benefit those suffering from many different types of cancers, including Wilms Tumours and Bartholin Gland Carcinoma. The following people have first-hand experience in the healing powers of this extraordinary plant.

Case Study #51: 13-Year-Old in Remission from Aggressive Soft Tissue Cancer Thanks to Cannabis

"Chico Ryder was 11 years old when he was diagnosed with Stage III/Group III parameningeal embryonal rhabdomyosarcoma, an especially aggressive soft tissue cancer, in December 2012. He began the long road to recovery and immediately began chemotherapy after diagnosis.

From February to March 2013, Chico completed a 28-session protocol of radiation, which consisted of one session a day, five days a week. The intense combination of these treatments caused horrendous side effects, including near-daily vomiting and painful nerve damage. It got so bad that every time Chico had chemotherapy, he needed to stay in the hospital.

Chico's parents, Paul and Angela Ryder, knew they needed to do something to mitigate the damage from conventional treatments, as well as boost their cancer-fighting power. Angela learned about cannabis oil, and they decided it was the right thing to do.

Chico had tried Marinol, a synthetic form of THC, which was somewhat effective at first but eventually lost potency. He began receiving whole plant cannabis oil from Aunt Zelda's collective in July 2013.

The impact of cannabis extract therapy was remarkable. While it did not fully reverse the side effects of the large doses of chemotherapy and radiation, there were significant improvements; Chico's vomiting reduced by half and the neuropathy stopped progressing. By August 2013, he was able to get off intravenous nutrition and begin using a g-tube, which is better for the liver.

The doctors also pushed a substantial amount of opiates on Chico, including methadone; cannabis oil was very effective at helping Chico get off these opiates. In addition, Chico's white blood cell counts recovered faster than expected after chemotherapy sessions, and he did not need to delay chemotherapy at all once he began using cannabis oil.

"I wish we had done it from the beginning. I believe cannabis oil helped the chemotherapy do its job and protected Chico's body from damage," said Angela.

Indeed, tetrahydrocannabinol (THC) has been proven to induce programmed cell death in rhabdomyosarcoma cells. Both THC and cannabidiol (CBD) are neuropro-tective antioxidants that help prevent neuropathy. Chico ingested ample amounts of THC and CBD during his treatment. At his peak, he was ingesting 900mg of THC and 500mg of CBD a day, using the respective THC-rich and CBD-rich strains.

In addition to cannabis, Chico had excellent nutrition and used an herbal formula designed to increase white blood cells.

Chico used a range of integrative therapies alongside the conventional treatment, including cannabis oil (which is legal in his home state of California), mistletoe, acupuncture, a range of supplements including medicinal mushrooms, IP6 and a whole host of others.

By November 2013, Chico was declared in remission. He has been able to drastically reduce his cannabis dose to 85mg of THC and 100mg of CBD a day. Chico has since recovered from much of the damage he endured, but there is still a fair way to go.

Chico continues to use these integrative therapies to help prevent relapse and is committed to helping spread the word, particularly about the benefits for cancer patients of cannabis oil and is actively campaigning for it to be more widely available to all cancer patients.

In fact, Chico has been instrumental in kickstarting discussion about a potential research project involving cannabis and paediatric cancer at UCLA where he was treated. Chico has lost too many friends to this monster of a disease to sit back and do nothing. He loves music, learning to play the drums and playing the latest video games. It is hopeful that with continued nutrition and cannabis extract therapy, Chico will completely recover."

Source: https://illegallyhealed.com/13-year-old-chico-ryder-is-kickin-cancer-with-cannabis-oil

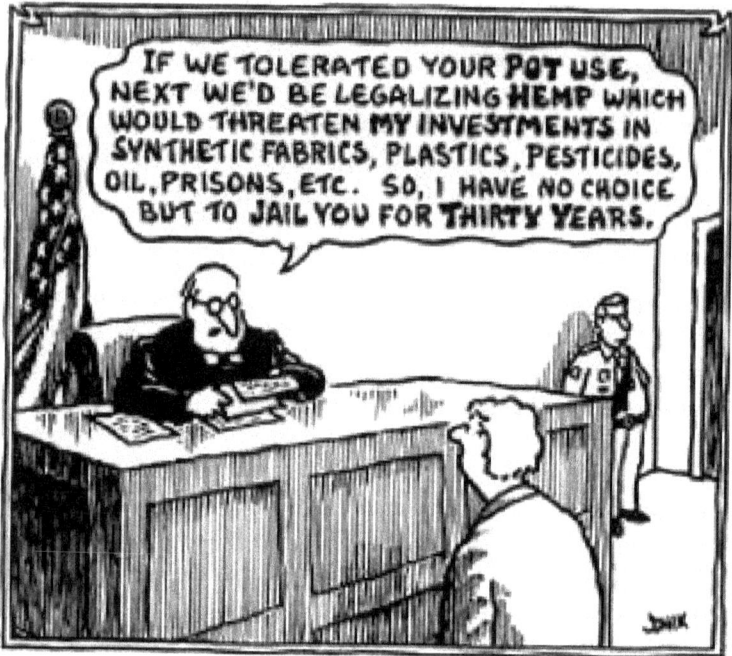

Case Study #52: Bartholin Gland Carcinoma...
Doctors Had Given Up

"A 47-year-old woman from Colorado said that Doctors had given up on her. She was diagnosed with Bartholin Gland Carcinoma and was taking a myriad of medications including Coumadin, Fentanyl, Lexapro, Lyrica, Neurotin, Percocet, Phenergan, and Xanax. Now, she's drug-free and in remission:

"I'm off all pharmaceuticals, cancer is gone, circulation has improved, and I was taken off the amputation list.

I took both THC and CBD, administered at 1000mg per day. Topical anointing oil for pain. I took five capsules in the morning and five capsules in the evening. It only took three weeks to kill the cancer.

I will never do chemo or radiation again. I have had 63 surgeries now thanks to the awful side effects. **Cannabis is the answer.**"

Source: www.cannabisoilsuccessstories.com/bartholin-gland-carcinoma--squamous-cell-.html

Case Study #53: Liver Mets Are Clear; 'Suspicious' Lungs Clear; Blood Pressure Perfect

"I started Full Extract Cannabis Oil about two months after diagnosis. I didn't know anything about dosing but started researching. Had high blood pressure, pre-diabetic, unbelievable pain from broken back.

The Cannabis Oil gave me instant relief from the pain. My left hip was breaking due to metastasis, so I had radiation on my hip and took Cannabis Oil starting the third day of treatment and daily thereafter during radiation. The first two days of radiation I was exhausted, burnt, nauseous and no appetite. After starting Cannabis Oil, I had no bad side effects. **Liver mets are clear! Cloudy 'suspicious' lungs are clear! Blood Pressure is perfect!** Blood sugar levels are perfect! I'm still here after 3.5 years!

Unfortunately, in the beginning a friend made my Cannabis Oil and we didn't know about testing. It was very high THC, I believe, and fueled the bone Metastasis and made Tamoxifen useless. I switched to a higher CBD Cannabis Oil (7:1 ratio) and the Metastasis stopped. I then switched to a 4:1 CBD-to-THC and am now on a 2:1 CBD-to-THC Oil.

For the first four months I took 1.25 grams per day. Both orally and suppositories. Liver cleared and metastasis stopped growing so I cut back to 1/10th of a gram orally per day. Stopped too soon and metastasis started to reappear. Now doing fifth of a gram orally per day. Take CBD oil in late afternoon, THC oil 3 hours later.

I'm still here! Can't say much more than that LOL. **I have good quality of life and am thankful for every day. Cannabis is helping save and extend my life.**"

Source: www.cannabisoilsuccessstories.com/aggressive-invasive-ductal-carcinoma.html

Case Study #54: 20-Year-Old Diagnosed With Mucoepidermoid Carcinoma... Sent Home To Die, Now Cancer Free

"In 2011 I was diagnosed with Stage II Hodgkin's Lymphoma that started in my chest then travelled to my neck. I had eight months of BEACOPP Chemotherapy (Bleomycin, Etoposide, Adriamycin, Cyclophosphamide, Oncovin-Vincristine, Procarbazine & Prednisone). At the end of my chemo I had 2.5 weeks of daily radiation therapy. I was in remission for 4.5 years.

In April 2016 I found a lump in my submandibular region (salivary gland) which was diagnosed as Mucoepidermoid carcinoma, a result of having radiation therapy in 2011. I had surgery to remove 30 lymph nodes, the tumour, one saliva gland and tissue from my neck. I then had six weeks of radiation therapy. Two weeks after radiation therapy I found a new lump, had it biopsied and it came back as the same cancer, Mucoepidermoid Carcinoma.

When they PET scanned me they found it had already spread to the other side of my neck. They said the only option was an enormous surgery where I would have a double neck dissection, the floor of my mouth removed, skin and muscle graft taken from my thigh muscle, the nerve that controls my tongue removed, the nerve that controls my bottom lip removed and a permanent breathing and feeding tube inserted. I refused this surgery and turned to Cannabis Oil. They sent me home to die and linked me to palliative care.

On November 30th, **after 13 weeks of taking Cannabis Oil, I was told I am in remission.** There was no evidence of tumours or cancerous activity.

Cannabis saved my life. I would not be here without it. I had never heard of this treatment as it is illegal here in Australia and only came across it as someone mentioned me to someone else who was using the oil. They got me in touch with the supplier and I went from there. **There is no doubt in my mind that this plant is a miracle drug and it should be legalized for medicinal use.** We could eradicate cancer completely! I am much less scared of cancer now because I know we are able to beat it with this God given plant."

Source: www.cannabisoilsuccessstories.com/mucoepidermoid-carcinoma--20-yo-female.html

Case Study #55: Cecilia's Story (Wilms Tumour)

"Our daughter Cecilia was diagnosed with Wilms Tumour on April 5, 2013 just before her 2nd birthday. Of course, we were devastated, but the doctors assured us because of having a low risk tumour with favourable histology and still only being stage 1 that with the regular protocol of chemotherapy she would have a 96% survival rate. So, she went through surgery to remove her right kidney along with a 2.5-pound tumour. She then underwent 20 weeks of chemotherapy.

Tragically, only five months later on February 28th, 2014 she relapsed with complete metastasis covering and collapsing her right lung. At the time, she needed a chest tube to remove the blood and fluid that had filled her chest cavity. She then had to begin eight rounds of radiation therapy to both lungs and underwent a much stronger and lengthy chemotherapy, but after only eight weeks into treatment her liver enzymes became dangerously high, causing her to miss over two months of treatment. With no other options other than experimental chemotherapy with no real statistics and no guarantee to her liver, we as parents made the difficult decision to leave the treatment and treat her 100% holistically.

At the end of April 2014, **Cecilia started using a combination of both CBD and THC Cannabis Oils** from Myriam's Hope, a medical Cannabis collective in southern California. Of course, we were scared but hopeful cannabis would help our daughter beat this disease. Before we left conventional treatment, we had a CT scan of her lungs still showing **three nodules measuring at 4.2mm, 8mm and 1.62mm.** In October, just three months later, we had another scan to make sure nothing was growing and incredibly she had over 3mm of shrinkage, the 8mm was now 5mm, the 4.2mm was less than 2mm and the 1.62mm could no longer be seen.

She has continued on Myriam's Hope Cannabis Oils and not only has she remained cancer-free, but she has gained close to ten pounds and lives a very active happy life of a regular 5-year-old child! We truly believe without Cannabis Oil we would not have our daughter with us today, not only did it save her life but helped her regain her health a vigour and give her the quality of life she deserves!"

Source: https://myriamshope.org/2016/06/i-have-completely-weaned-myself-off-of-all-pharmaceuticals-thanks-to-myriams-hope

CHAPTER 14

Epilepsy, Seizures, and Cannabis

In America alone, 3 million people are affected by epilepsy and seizures, and every year brings about 200,000 additional cases. According to a study published in 2013, premature death is eleven times more common among epilepsy patients. Cannabis can bring real hope to these patients.

Case Study #56: 5-year-old Katelyn Lambert Miraculously Improves Using Cannabis

"An Australian philanthropist has donated $3 million to fund medical marijuana research at the Lambert Center for the Study of Medicinal Cannabis at Thomas Jefferson University in Philadelphia, Pennsylvania.

70-year-old Barry Lambert earned a substantial fortune as the founder of Count Financial, Australia's biggest accounting firm support network. He has a history of donating generously to various causes, but in this case, Lambert's motivation is rather personal.

His 5-year-old granddaughter Katelyn, who suffers from a rare form of epilepsy called Dravet syndrome, displayed "miraculous" improvement after being treated with cannabis oil. After witnessing such dramatic relief from the seizures and other symptoms associated with the condition, Lambert became interested in backing cannabis research.

The Aussie businessman says he has had no previous experience with marijuana but believes in its promise in treating a number of illnesses. "It's about doing the right thing," Lambert told the *Australian Financial Review*. "There are all these uses for cannabis but, because it's illegal, it's never been researched."

In fact, Lambert has already contributed $34 million to the University of Sydney to fund a program called the Lambert Initiative for Cannabinoid Therapeutics:

"The Lambert Initiative has been established with a wide mission to investigate a range of possible applications: epilepsy; stimulating appetite in chemotherapy patients; tremors from multiple sclerosis; pain relief for the terminally ill; treatment of addiction and post-traumatic stress disorder."

Lambert and his wife Joy's decision to also fund cannabis research at Thomas Jefferson University was inspired by "Jefferson's rapid progress in the field of medicinal cannabis research and innovative approach to exploring all avenues for new therapies to include using hemp-derived cannabinoids," he said in a press release.

Joy Lambert played a key role in the family's decision to explore cannabis as a possible treatment for her grand-daughter. When Katelyn's father Michael began researching cannabis as a treatment option, Joy suppor-ted his efforts. Before Katelyn began her cannabis oil therapy, **she was barely able to speak**, and suffered from frequent and painful seizures. "It's like watching your child being electrocuted to death," said Michael.

Shortly after a "trial and error" phase when Michael first began administering cannabis oil to Katelyn, the child began showing a marked improvement, with her seizures becoming far less frequent and shorter in duration. Katelyn began regaining her ability to speak, and in many respects, now leads a normal life. "She is a person now," Michael said. "She is well."

[...] With millions invested in marijuana research, Barry Lambert has single-handedly performed a great deed for humanity. Medicinal marijuana research may benefit millions of people in the future, thanks to the vision and generosity of Lambert and others who are determined to "do the right thing."

Source: www.naturalnews.com/2016-12-14-australian-philanthropist-donated-millions-for-medical-marijuana-research-after-it-miraculously-helped-treat-his-granddaughters-ep.html

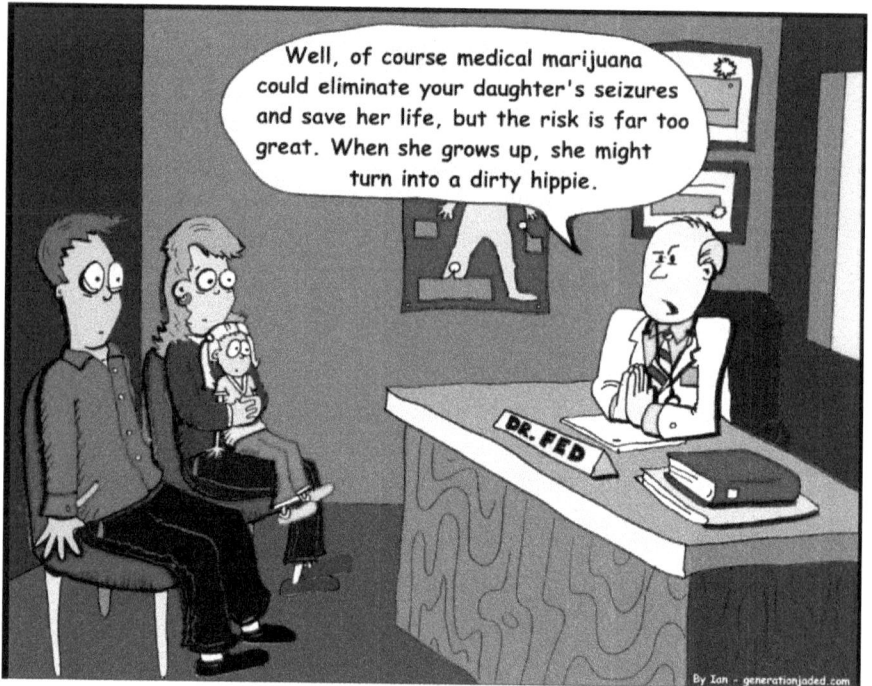

By Ian - generationjaded.com

Case Study #57: Annalise Lujan's Battle with Life-Threatening Seizures

"Earlier this year, 12-year-old girl Annalise Lujan was competing in a Tucson gymnastics competition when she started vomiting and lost all feeling in her legs. By her fourth event, she just couldn't move. She couldn't walk. She just was exhausted, tired, not feeling well," Maryann Estrada-Lujan, Annalise's mother told KVOA.

When her parents took her to the Banner University Medical Center (UMC) in Tucson, Annalise was diagnosed with a stomach bug and sent home. The next night, however, she had her first seizure. Concerned about the health of their daughter, Annalise's parents took her back to the UMC. Again, she was sent home without further treatment. The next morning her condition deteriorated quickly, with the girl being plagued by more seizures.

As her parents rushed her to the hospital, the 12-year-old fell into a crippling seizure. According to her mom, she was put on life support and was put into an induced coma to save her brain from damage. Two and a half weeks later she was airlifted to Phoenix Children's Hospital, where doctors diagnosed her with an extremely rare epilepsy syndrome called Febrile Infection-Related Epilepsy Syndrome (FIRES).

As noted by Annalise's dad, only one in a million children will get this syndrome. Experts believe that this little-understood condition occurs after an ordinary cold or stomach virus spreads to the brain or autoimmune system. It usually starts two weeks after a child has had a mild fever then quickly gets worse until patients have seizures continuously, with some children having up to 100 seizures a day. Since these constant seizures can lead to brain injury and death, doctors had to put her into an induced coma.

Annalise came out of the coma after less than 48-hours of CBD treatment.

To bring her back to the living, doctors had to find a way to control the seizures. Unfortunately, regular anti-epilepsy drugs don't work on this extremely rare condition. This prompted Annelise's mother to research other, alternative ways to save her daughter's life.

During her search, she stumbled on a cannabis-derived drug, called cannabidiol or CBD oil. Unlike Rick Simpson's hemp oil, which is known for its cancer-fighting properties, CBD oil has very low levels of THC, which is the substance that creates the cannabis high.

With the substance not being approved at that time and no other route to take, Annalise's doctors had to rush CBD's approval through the FDA and DEA. Currently, cannabis for both medical and recreational use is legal in

Colorado, Washington, Alaska, Oregon, Nevada, Maine, California, and Massachusetts.

Less than 48 hours after her first CBD oil treatment, the 12-year-old was cured of the constant seizures and opened her eyes.

"She opened her eyes, and she was scared. She was afraid. She cried. And, I whispered to her that she's beautiful, she's strong, and she needs to keep breathing, and she did," Maryann said.

Although Annalise remains in the hospital for further recovery and to regain the cognitive functions she had before, cannabidiol oil has saved this little girl's life.

While experts don't want to call it a cure, because patients must keep taking it daily to prevent seizures, CBD oil offers hope for nearly three million Americans who suffer from epilepsy. For a third of these people, standard epilepsy drugs do not work to control their symptoms. They may even do more harm than good.

Though there is still a lot of controversy surrounding the medical use of marijuana, more people are discovering its amazing healing effects."

Source: www.naturalnews.com/2017-06-08-cannabis-oil-cbd-cures-12-year-old-girl-of-life-threatening-seizures.html

Case Study #58: Baby Suffers 300 Seizures a Week

"When Nicole and Ernie Nunez brought their few-days-old daughter, Amylea, to the hospital in New Mexico, no one could identify the source of her seizures. As her parents grew desperate with the idleness of her doctors, they decided to look for an alternative cure. What they found was the high-CBD cannabis oil called Charlotte's

Web, which may have saved their daughter's life.

When Amylea was born in December, her parents were absolutely thrilled to bring her home. Only a few hours later, however, everything went wrong as Amylea suffered her first seizure. Her parents rushed her to the hospital, but the doctors were unable to pinpoint the source. Desperate with the situation, Nicole and Ernie Nunez took Amylea to the Children's Hospital in Aurora, Colorado, where she has already spent the first two months of her life.

The situation was no better here than in New Mexico, however. As doctors tried all kinds of medications on young Amylea, she continued to suffer from seizures. While her mother spent all of her time by her side, Ernie ran back and forth between the hospital and their home in Albuquerque. The medication prescribed to Amylea was known to be especially taxing on her frail two-month-old liver, so her parents were determined to find a better treatment.

It seemed that, at this point, doctors could do nothing more than stand helplessly and watch Amylea's condition worsen. **It was up to Nicole to do the research and come up with an alternative.**

Once Nicole started looking for natural remedies for epilepsy, she came across the cannabis oil known as Charlotte's Web. This miraculous strain of cannabis was named after an American girl who suffered from Dravet syndrome as a baby. Her name was Charlotte Figi, and she too was experiencing severe epilepsy like Amylea. By the time she was three, Charlotte was seriously disabled. In spite of treatment, she was experiencing approximately 300 seizures every week.

Her parents looked beyond conventional medicine and found a strain of marijuana that could be used for treatment. They began immediately and saw vast improvement. With a regular regimen using the high-CBD cannabis extract, Charlotte was finally able to engage in normal childhood activities. Now, she only experienced about four seizures a month.

Nicole Nunez saw hope in Charlotte's story and immediately proposed this alternative treatment to Amylea's doctors. For weeks, they refused to proceed with the treatment. Earlier in February, however, the doctors finally agreed to Nicole's solution and the parents began treating their daughter with Charlotte's Web. **After only two doses, both Amylea's parents and her doctors could notice the difference. The oil had worked.**

Amylea's story is a glimmer of hope for those infants struggling with epilepsy."

Source: www.naturalnews.com/054285_cannabis_oil_CBD_epilepsy.html

Case Study #59: 30 Grand Mal Seizures A Day Reduced To Zero With Cannabis

"My son was diagnosed with epilepsy at the age of six months, having up to 30 grand mal seizures a month.

He has been one year seizure-free since he was completely weaned off pharmaceuticals, on December 17, 2016. **We use CBD tinctures with less than 0.03% THC.** We give my son three droppers of CBD tincture per day [one dropper is 10mg of CBD].

When this journey started I was a mom and my second child developed epilepsy. We were in and out of the hospital, doctors trying to give multiple medications to my baby. We started him on Keppra and he was still having multiple seizures a day, some days. And yet all of his tests came back 'normal'. We couldn't find an answer.

126

I was at the hospital while my son was having an EEG test and a young couple were talking about Cannabis Oil and I asked them if they had any information. They did, and while I was sitting, watching my baby boy going through this I knew I had to do something! At our next doctor visit my son's neurologist asked me 'do you think Keppra is working?' and my response was 'NO!!!' So he said let's go with CBD oil only.

It took eight weeks total to wean him off the Keppra. **In the first 30 days he only had one seizure! I was shocked!** I kept weaning him and his last seizure was December 17, 2015 and the last day of him taking Keppra was December 18, 2015. He's still on CBD oil and he's doing amazing!"

Source: www.cannabisoilsuccessstories.com/epilepsy--grand-mal-seizures--1.html

Case Study #60: Atlanta Now Seizure Free Thanks To Cannabis Extracts

"Hello, my name is Atlanta and I have epilepsy from being a shaken baby. I actually attended a CBD event in my hometown at a friend's house where they talked about all the benefits CBD had for all kinds of issues. I told them my story and what all I had going on and they advised me to try it. I was shaken when I was three months old and was on life support. Out of an act of God I came back from that with epilepsy and a Ventriculoperitoneal shunt in my head to drain fluid out of my brain.

Nine months later I was able to have the shunt removed but I had a serious scar on my head.

The first ten years of my life I went through so many medications and therapies and EEGs in the hospital I can't even count. We finally found a medication that worked; it was Tegratol and worked good for about two years, then it threw me into massive amounts of catatonic seizures.

A guy from Hawaii sought me out and had me try his THCA oil and **it literally changed my life. I haven't had any seizures for over three months.** I literally could feel a shock from the first taste of this THCA oil.

And there are so many more people that it has been able to help, so many testimonies and miracles. I tried two other oils and nothing compares to how THCA has changed my life. I would love to help more people like myself change their quality of life. **I am still seizure-free; a couple months ago I couldn't imagine this!**

We went on a vacation and I was able to have an amazing time because I had no more issues. I sleep better, I dream better I don't get light headed any more or have tracers. My headaches have decreased and I haven't had to get more injections for them. I am pharmaceutical free. AND I AM KICKING ASS!!!! Your life can be just as great and on top too."

Source: www.cannabisoilsuccessstories.com/epilepsy---insomnia---restless-leg-syndrome.html

Case Study #61: From 500+ Seizures Per Month to Zero Thanks To Cannabis Extracts

"At age nine, Donna was playing hide-and-seek at church one Sunday morning and was found having a seizure while hiding. As far back as she can remember, she has had daily seizure activity, upwards of 20 or more when no medication was available. She says:

"My epilepsy is considered intractable, meaning Western medicine doesn't have an effect on the seizure activity.

Prior to using Cannabis, I was prescribed a number of medications over the years, none of it helped to decrease the number of daily seizures; increasing the frequency and intensity instead of any therapeutic benefit whatsoever and the side-effects were very unpleasant. Everything from weight gain, allergic reactions, sleepiness, severe depression, postictal psychosis to failed suicide attempts. **I had no other choice to ditch the big pharma medications and give cannabis a try.**"

Donna was on the following medications with no benefits whatsoever: Dilantin, Depakote, Lacosamide, Lamotrigine (Lamictal), Levetira-cetam (Keppra), Tegretol.

Donna continues: "A loved one and I packed up all that could fit in a car, leaving Indiana and its obtrusive laws. Ending up in Portland Oregon, we struggled living in the car and eventually traded in for an RV eventually settling on the coastal area. My friend then contacted a Cannabis consultant for me, after reading an article online about a local Cannabis activist; someone who had apparent success treating a few patients of seizures. So, we set up an appointment and **from the first time I took the Cannabis extract, my life changed for the better...**"

The Cannabis extracts that have worked to curb Donna's seizures have all been primarily THC with very minimal amounts of CBD. The Cannabis concentrate is mixed with coconut oil and heated to create an infusion, typically dispensed from a dropper bottle so more accurate dosing can be administered.

Cannabis extract gel capsules were also implemented, and Donna can take one at night and not have any pre-seizure activity for the duration of the 24 hours between capsules, although she does administer a tincture or use a vaporizer at points throughout the day.

Donna began using approximately 12 drops of Cannabis-infused coconut oil when she felt the onset of seizure activity. This prevented any seizures from occurring, as long as she was able to take the medicine within minutes. The three seizures Donna had in the first two months of this method were due to her inability to access the medicine.

After two months, Donna went to a set schedule of taking 6 drops four times each day: upon waking, around noon, around 4 PM and once before bed. By keeping the Cannabis in her system, she didn't have any pre-seizure auras or other activity and she slept better than she had in years.

After three weeks of using Cannabis four times a day, Donna switched to taking one gel capsule, approximately 0.1 grams of concentrated Cannabis extract, just before bed. On the first night, she went 23.5 hours before feeling the need for more, so she adjusted and added a few drops of the coconut oil infusion around 10 PM and that protocol seems to carry her through to the next once-a-day Cannabis gel capsule she takes before bed each night.

Donna adds: "The pain of the grand mals and the post-seizure hallucinations sets off the depression and PTSD, leading me down the path of contemplating suicide and feeling helpless, being a constant burden to friends and family. The combination of cannabis oil and flower combats all of those problems and I can state without a doubt that **the Cannabis extracts are literally saving my life**."

Source: www.cannabisoilsuccessstories.com/epilepsy--donna-from-indiana.html

Case Study #62: Refractory General Epilepsy Stops Within Weeks Thanks To Cannabis

"Smoking Cannabis provided comfort but did little to cease the seizures. Recorded over 100 seizures in a 5-night sleep study (EMU) 2003 original DLBC diagnosis, treated conventionally, recurrence into Stage 4 low.

Twenty-seven medications were used from 1995-2013 to try to control severe refractory epilepsy (back-to-back grand mals, non-medically treatable, pills didn't work).

At the time of the initial CBD/Full extract use in Sept. 2013 I was on five AEDs, three Benzos, and pain medication. Since 9/8/2013 I have not had a grand mal seizure and no longer have a positive reading on EEG (Brain wave testing); **seizures moved quickly from severe to minor to none within the first weeks of treatment using Cannabis Oil.**

My Hodgkin's Nodular Lymphoma went into full remission within 90 days of the diagnosis in 2015, while my DLBC NHL has morphed to lesser forms of this radical growth type of Lymphoma. At first it metastisized into both the clavicle (collarbone) and into the brachial plexus (large nerve located below it) causing severe pain and flaring on PET exams, making it appear that Cancer was ongoing throughout 2016. Only now in December are they figuring out it's nerve metastasis that's going to take years to heal, if ever (nerve sheaths generally don't heal).

My choice to use Cannabis Oil wasn't an easy one to make. As a non-attorney representative for kids in special education disputes, I had to take a serious look at how my clients and the administrative law courts would react. The initial reaction was as I thought – not good at all. I was both thrown off cases and blocked or fired by parents that didn't want a 'pothead' to represent them.

Without Cannabis, I would be dead, as would many of my child clients, both in special education and in a compassion program I voluntarily direct. **It's our right to use nature and my life is a testimony that the use of nature over pills is the difference between living and existing; the difference between life and death.** I used to read stories about people with cancer getting better and wonder if they were true, and now I'm a walking success story; **daily as I use Cannabis Oil and my oncologist watches in amazement as all tumour growth within lymph nodes has ceased and is gone.** Nine points of surgical concern in Nov 2015 are now NONE! Severe Epilepsy? **After 40 months of no Epileptic seizures, I often forget I even have it!** Those days are over... The seizure days are over."

Source: www.cannabisoilsuccessstories.com/refractory-generalized-epilipsy.html

Case Study #63: Intractable Epileptic Encephalopathy Treated With Cannabis Extracts

"[Before Cannabis Extract]: hundreds of Myoclonic seizures per day; tonic 1 to 4 Clonic seizures per week and atypical Absence 5-10/week. Very drowsy, sleeping 16-18 hours per day with constant drooling.

There were sensory processing issues; he did a lot of clapping and banging on his legs to self-stimulate Also, very poor conversational skills. He couldn't hold a conversation past the initial "what are you doing" question.

He finished Second Grade only knowing half of the alphabet, couldn't sound any letters out or spell any words, couldn't participate in group discussions in class as he could not grasp the concept of contributing like ideas and thoughts.

He had status seizures every 2-3 months which resulted in Emergency Room trips and 4-7-day hospital stays; to the PICU half the time. Too weak from seizures and medications to use most playground equipment (anything that required upper body strength) and 8-10 second delays between hearing a question and actually processing it to respond.

[After Cannabis Extracts]: "Seizure-free since April 2016, aside from a handful of seizures while weaning and adjusting medications. He rarely naps during the day, most days he only sleeps about 12 hours. **He has stopped drooling, stopped banging on the walls, the clapping/leg slapping has been reduced by about 90% and he can have a conversation** with about 4-5 questions that he can recall.

Within one month of starting Third Grade, he knows his full alphabet, the sounds for all of his letters, a word for each letter and can spell half a dozen words. He also now understands the concept of numbers and how they relate to counting objects/money and can contribute simple ideas to group discussions.

We haven't been to the ER since the day we started [cannabis] oil, he can hold his own weight on the monkey bars for about half of the way across, and now has just a 4-5 second delay in response.

Dosing is 20mg/ml of CBD 1mg/ml of THC per dropper, and he takes two droppers [1ml each] in the morning and in the evening. Total per dosing is 40mg of CBD and 2mg THC, so a daily total of 80mg CBD and 4mg THC.

Cannabis has changed our lives. I feel like I am meeting the bright, funny, silly boy he used to be before he had seizures. He used to be advanced for his age at all of his check-ups, until he began having seizures. Since seizures and medications, he had fallen behind so far developmentally. I have missed out on experiencing the milestones all parents look forward to. He has missed out on a normal childhood. He has grown up in hospitals and consumed gallons and gallons of medications that have done so much damage.

Cannabis has given us the control that drugs never could, at a fraction of the dose and without any of the side effects that pharmaceuticals gave him. **I finally have hope that he can catch up developmentally and be seizure free** and able to get a driver's license down the road. We have already weaned off of Vimpat and will begin weaning off Divalproex in the new year!"

Source: www.cannabisoilsuccessstories.com/intractable-epileptic-encephalopathy.html

Case Study #64: Lennox-Gastaut Syndrome: I Am Beginning To See My Daughter Again

"Diana started having seizures as a new-born at 9 days old; she is now 19. She was sedated, locked in her own shell. We have tried at least 14 different anti-epileptic medications, given in different combinations, most recently Banzal, Keppra, Lamictal, Lamotrigine, Onfi [still on 10mg/day] and Vimpat.

This has been a long journey; we started Cannabis in December of 2013. **Since starting the extracts, all seizures are under a minute long with no Postictal state.** She has increased eye contact and is aware of her surroundings and those around her. She is laughing at appropriate times, watching her sisters, and the dog. We were able to wean her off three anti-epileptic medications with the help of THCa.

We give a low dose of CBD with terpenes, under 25 mg as more makes her stimming behaviours worse. Also THC-a, THC, CBN with terpenes. We give one dose of CBD per day, two doses of THCa, and a dose of CBN a half-hour before bed. If needed, we will give a dose of THC for breakthrough seizures 20-35 mg depending on the seizure type.

I am beginning to see my daughter again, since being on the seizure medications she was lost! She now has eye contact and looks around at everything. She is a teenager and can be stubborn. She is also starting to be more vocal, I haven't heard her voice since she was 2 1/2 years old, the sounds are coming!"

Source: www.cannabisoilsuccessstories.com/lennox-gastaut-syndrome--lgs-.html

Case Study #65: Two-Year-Old Ava Barry Experienced More Than 400 Seizures a Month

"Our little girl, Ava, was diagnosed in 2010 with Dravet Syndrome, a rare and intractable form of epilepsy, described as drug-resistant. It involves severe development delay and uncontrolled seizures.

Ava was experiencing daily seizures which included hundreds of absent seizures, staring spells, and myoclonic jerks where her limbs would jerk involuntarily, and she experienced tonic clonic seizures almost every day. The unpredictable nature of Dravet Syndrome meant Ava could have more than a dozen tonic clonic seizures some days and on other days she would have maybe one or two; these violent seizures could last from between two minutes or up to an hour or longer on occasion. Ava would have absence seizures and myo jerks alongside these tonic clonic seizures, resulting in more than four or five hundred seizures every month.

At about two years old, Ava experienced a week-long coma following a number of seizures. She had just learned to walk at this time and we were incredibly proud of her. The seizures resulted in her losing the ability to walk and it took another twelve months before she walked again. The coma also robbed her of her first word which was "nice" and she didn't say the word for another eighteen months. Ava made her way through eleven different anti-epilepsy medications before we were told in October 2015 that no other medication was available to help Ava. We asked doctors what we do now, and they said "take her home." I became frantic and asked them "home to what." They replied, "there is no more medication, we have tried everything."

We began a Facebook page "CBD For Ava Support". Please do feel free to visit the page, or my own page Vera Twomey.

In November 2015, **Ava had a heart attack after eighteen seizures in nine hours.** Again, our daughter nearly lost her life, it was another horrifying experience. I will never forget the journey to the hospital from home where I had returned just a few hours earlier. Collected by a close relative we raced to the hospital and received a call on the way from Ava's doctor to hurry, we needed to get there fast. On arrival I discovered my husband in pieces, crying, and I thought seeing him in this condition, that Ava had passed away, but again the steel in my daughter came to the fore and she fought back like many other parents have seen their children do.

She recovered and thank God we brought her home, and 2016 continued with seizures, ear infections, colds, seizures, ear infections, seizures, then no infections at all, then more seizures, and beyond that more seizures; we had no hope.

To get medicinal Cannabis we contacted political people, radio stations, and TV in an effort to access medical Cannabis for Ava. We had meetings with government officials, however progress was slow. In September of 2016 we were made aware that Charlotte's Web was becoming available in Ireland, so we went to Dublin and purchased a bottle. After more than four years of research into medical Cannabis, we were still worried we would do the wrong thing for Ava but at the end of September, **Ava suffered twenty-three seizures in thirty-six hours and we decided that CBD was our next option.**

Since beginning Charlotte's Web in October of 2016, Ava has had seven seizures in October, nine in November, five in December, and three in January of 2017. **She has not been admitted to the hospital once since she began Charlotte's Web,** nor has she needed bucel Midas since October. She has not had to be put on oxygen and we have had no visit from ambulance she is speaking more standing better walking better her school has noted the improvement in concentration her appetite has improved and what I feel is very important she is smiling more and able to play more with her two younger sisters and brother who also adore her.

We give Ava Charlotte's Web CBD extract. Our decision to use it was related to Charlotte Figi's success with it. Ava gets Charlotte's Web twice a day; morning and evening. The dose is based on her weight, and we were helped with getting correct dosage for Ava via the Realm of Caring website and The Hemp Store on Capel street in Dublin where we purchased the oil for Ava.

Cannabis in a medicinal form has given my daughter, Ava Barry, the opportunity to have a life that is not ruled or controlled by epilepsy. It has given my daughter an opportunity to see the world without pain, without holding her body because her muscles ache. It has given her the chance to let the wonderful person that she is shine through. Her smile is broad and her eyes exhibit more understanding and liveliness. Cannabis has reduced the terrible fear that was palpable in our home. We can now arrange little trips to Macroom or Cork without as much fear that Ava will have a seizure. It has allowed our other children to have their sister to themselves without having to worry about Ava going to the hospital for "big medicine" as Ava's sisters and brother are all five and under the ongoing interruption of hospital oxygen masks ambulances and seizures are now not as much a feature of our lives.

Cannabis has set our family free, allowed us to begin a new type of life where we know of course Ava's condition is not cured, but Cannabis has given Ava such a significant improved life that all the people around her have an element of enjoyment that was sadly absent before. Cannabis has altered our lives and I truly hope a day comes when other families faced with the same condition or similar will not have to fight so hard to get a medicine for their small child that really works."

Source: www.cannabisoilsuccessstories.com/dravet-syndrome--7-yo-female.html

CHAPTER 15

Autism and Cannabis

Medical professionals have a consensus that there is no known 'cure' for autism. However, the following 4 testimonials I'm going to share with you will open your eyes to the incredible benefits of cannabis oil for children with Autism.

Case Study #66: Kalel Santiago Starts Talking After Only Two Days on CBD Oil

"CBD oil (Cannabidiol) has long been proven to combat negative effects of numerous health problems. Of course, due to the fact that it isn't being peddled by the drug-pushing pharmaceutical companies, this information has been kept out of the hands of the average American citizen. Instead, they are still being led to believe that anything related to cannabis and marijuana is evil and should never be consumed.

Unfortunately for them, the facts don't support their ridiculous claims. In fact, they completely disregard them.

139

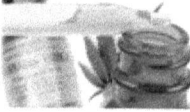

Consider Kalel Santiago — a **three-year-old boy in Puerto Rico suffering from severe autism**. After years of not speaking, Kalel was given CBD oil, and **after just two days of use, began talking to his parents.**

The Free Thought Project reports, "Kalel's parents knew very little about autism at the time and sought out a way to ensure that their child would be helped. They found measurable success from various schools and therapeutic techniques including one that used surfing as a means of therapy. After trying various methods, the Santiago family was made aware of Cannabidiol (CBD) oil as a non-psychoactive treatment for autism."

People like **Kalel Santiago benefit tremendously from CBD oil, without causing any harm**, so how can the federal government in the United States justify keeping it from people like him?"

Source: https://eraoflight.com/2016/10/24/cannabis-oil-helps-autistic-boy-finally-speak-after-only-2-days-of-use

Case Study #67: Autism Outlook Much Brighter Thanks to Cannabis Extracts

"My 6-year-old daughter often seemed in her own world. She had a hard time focusing on non-preferred activities. She would run from us at places where she became overstimulated, like parking lots, theme parks and grocery stores. She was extremely rigid with her schedule and would have a meltdown if things didn't go the way she expected. She spoke in mostly one to two-word phrases with no conversational skills whatsoever. She was beginning to get aggressive and would target her teachers, aides, babysitter and little sister almost daily. She was a picky eater, eating only a few foods. She would wake up 2-3 times a week at 1-2 AM and stay awake the rest of the night. She would verbal stim constantly.

She is doing amazingly well [now she uses cannabis extract]. She's present with us like she's never been before. She can focus for longer periods of time on activities that are non-preferred. She can go to the grocery store with us now and instead of running down the aisles, she helps us push the cart and bag the groceries. **Her aggression is 100% gone.** She is using more sentences and speaking in longer 5-7-word phrases. We have conversations now, daily with two to four exchanges. She is eating more foods and even eating greens. She sleeps through the night and hasn't woken up once in the middle of the night since starting cannabis. She is more flexible with her schedule, has less anxiety and has better control of her emotions. Her verbal stimming is becoming less and less.

We started with 3:1 CBD:THC. I got ACDC and OG Kush oils from Myriam's Hope and mixed them myself. After a month I noticed the CBD:THC not being as effective and through some trial and error and research, we switched to 1:1 THC-A:THC, and the results have been amazing. Currently using THC-A from OG Kush (Myriam's Hope) and THC from Girl Scout Cookie (Cannakids). I have several mixes/ratios of these oils that I rotate around depending on how my daughter is doing. If you mix the strains regularly, we have noticed (and we learned this from other autism parents) that the oils remain effective for longer periods of time.

Dosing Schedule: "With CBD:THC we used 2.5 mg THC and 7.5 mg CBD at morning, afternoon and night. With THC-A:THC we used 2 mg THC with 2 mg of THC-A. I give her a glass of mango juice to wash it down which I believe helps with keeping the doses low as the permeability of the blood brain barrier is increased by the terpenes in mangos.

I used to have no clue what my daughter's future would look like. Getting the autism diagnosis when she was three years old, our dreams for her were shattered. We didn't know if she'd ever talk or if she'd go to college or if she'd even have a normal relationship with anyone. Now our hope is restored. She's doing so well we now have hope for her future again. **There is a light at the end of this autism tunnel where before it was hard to find**. We believe she'll lead a fairly normal life with some support (and Cannabis)."

Source: www.cannabisoilsuccessstories.com/autism-outlook-positive-with-cannabis.html

Case Study #68: Benjamin's Story

"It's morning in Nahariya, a tiny Israeli town near the Lebanese border, and 4-year-old Benjamin is repeatedly smashing his head against the wall. He spins wildly in circles, screeching at full volume. As his mother tries frantically to calm him, he pulls down his pants and defecates on the floor.

When they leave their apartment, Benjamin wrestles free of her hand and nearly runs into oncoming traffic. Sharon attempts a trip to the supermarket but leaves before she finishes shopping because her son is screaming while he picks up items and throws them to the floor.

That was in October 2016, and typical of most days at the time. Sharon, a single mother who moved to Israel from the United States one year earlier, was alone and losing control. Benjamin was taking Ritalin, a drug usually associated with attention deficit hyperactivity disorder (ADHD), which he did not have. He'd also tried the antipsychotic ziprasidone and a mix of antidepressants and anti-anxiety drugs. None of them helped, and he often became more hyperactive as they wore off.

All that changed a year ago, when Benjamin started taking cannabis. In the little apartment he shares with his mother, mornings are now relaxed and orderly. His transformation may signal the arrival of a long-awaited and desperately needed healing for the many others just like him: children living with severe autism.

[...] By October 2016, Sharon was desperate. She gave birth to Benjamin alone and chose to move to Israel to be part of a close-knit community. But his condition was isolating. She was lost, alone, exhausted, frustrated. More than all that, she was sad for her child.

One day, while filling Benjamin's regular prescription for Ritalin, Sharon vented about the side effects to the pharmacist. He responded with a surprising suggestion. She should contact Dr. Adi Aran, he said, a paediatric neurologist in Jerusalem who had begun experimenting with medical cannabis as a treatment for children like Benjamin.

Sharon balked at first. Benjamin wasn't even in first grade. And wasn't marijuana a dangerous and illegal drug? But at the same time, she had tried every option that conventional medicine had to offer. In other words, she had nothing to lose.

In Israel, cannabis use is legal in a small number of medical cases, such as epilepsy, severe chronic pain and certain forms of cancer. Aran, who directs the paediatric neurology unit at Jerusalem's Shaare Zedek hospital, had been recommending cannabis for some of the epileptic children he treated. At the end of 2015, he began an informal study of medical cannabis for severe autism.

In online forums for parents of children with ASD, Sharon read about some new forms of cannabis that were created specifically for young children. **She watched an Israeli documentary from that year that showed children with ASD transformed by medical marijuana.** The more she learned, the more determined she became to enroll Benjamin in the Israeli study. She sent Aran an email begging him to consider treating him, and he invited the mother and son to Jerusalem.

It was a fraught trip. The five-hour journey, by bus and train, included several violent outbursts and meltdowns. At the hospital, Aran reviewed Benjamin's medical history and observed his behaviour. Seeing the severity of his symptoms and the long list of medications that had already been tried without success, the doctor agreed that he was a good candidate. Sharon was sent home with a prescription for an oil made from a specially calibrated strain of Israeli cannabis, along with paperwork to chart her son's progress.

[...] Within two weeks of filling the prescription from Aran, Sharon says, he was calmer. He responded when she spoke to him. He could sit still and make eye contact. If she took him with her to visit friends, she could sit with the adults drinking tea while he played quietly in the other room. **Within months, he was doing so well that his teachers recommended he leave his special-needs school for a standard classroom**. "It's like a miracle. I can leave the house and go out with him and not worry," says Sharon. "I can breathe."

144

[...] In the meantime, Aran stresses the need to change the anti-marijuana stigma that still pervades American medicine and drug regulation. "Giving marijuana to children is unthinkable, but CBD is not marijuana," he says. "It's not a drug. It's a medication."

Source: https://uk.news.yahoo.com/marijuana-world-most-effective-treatment-130002295.html

Case Study #69: I Give My 7 Year Old Son Cannabis Oil to Treat His Autism

"We started to think about giving him meds about a year or so ago. The catalyst is he was getting incredibly violent (hitting us, his brother, the dog), wouldn't settle down to sleep even though we have been giving him Melatonin. No amount of ABA or behavioural therapy seemed to work. So we met with an autism psychologist, and put him on anti-psychotic meds. I don't remember what he's gone through, but his currently on Risperdal. The effects have ranged from manic hyperness, to violent outbursts, etc.

The Rispradol works... ok. It mellowed him out a little bit, but not much. The possible side-effects are intense. He can grow boobs, his tongue can swell and affect his speech, etc. Triglycerides, prolactin can both go to unsafe levels without monitoring.

Basically, we were at our wits end. We wanted to help him and just give him the calm he needed, without the crazy side-effects of prescription meds. We did a TON of research, and thought it was the best option considering the circumstances. There is a doctor in Berkley that specialized in children cannabis therapy for autism and epilepsy. He thought it could help, so we went for it. This was a couple weeks ago, and the results have been pretty profound.

145

The first night we gave it to him, he went right to sleep. He usually spends about 30-45minutes yelling and hitting the wall. He's gone right to sleep every night since.

He says some things unprompted! Today he came up to me to get my attention and said my name! This is an absolute first.

He's just… happy. He has very few outbursts/fits, and when he does their fairly benign and end quickly.

He's taken to peeing on the patio…but that's good! Usually he'd just go in his diaper. But now he knows to stand and pee. Now we need to work on the right place to pee, but it's a start!

He looks in people's eyes MUCH more.

He can actually sit and attend to a task. The other day he tolerated a haircut for 15-20 minutes. I can't express how amazing this part is. This kid couldn't sit still for 2 minutes, but now he's tolerating a haircut? Which he HATES? We were flabbergasted.

My wife dropped him off at ABA the other day. He grabbed the therapist's hand, turned to my wife and said "Bye!", turned to the lady and said, "Let's go." and off he went. Usually ABA visits devolve into some sort of fit tantrum.

I know some of you might not agree with this treatment, especially a child, but I'm here to tell you it's working."

Source:www.reddit.com/r/autism/comments/3h9q30/i_give_my_son_who_is _7_cannabis_oil_to_treat_his

CHAPTER 16

Cerebral Palsy and Cannabis

Cerebral Palsy is one of the most common childhood disorders in the United States. Medical costs are around 10 times higher for children with this condition. But in this chapter, I share case studies of children with Cerebral Palsy whose lives have been transformed by using cannabis extracts.

Case Study #70: Relief from Cerebral Palsy is Just One Reason to Legalize Medical Cannabis

"Cerebral palsy (CP) is a neurological disorder caused by brain injury or abnormal development of the brain before, during, or immediately after birth. The effects of CP vary largely between individuals, but usually involve some type of movement dysfunction in the arms, legs, and/or face. While conventional treatments can help with symptoms, there is no cure.

Jacqueline Patterson is a well-known medical cannabis activist with mild spastic CP that affects the left side of her brain and right side of her body and has resulted in arthritis in her left hand. She has shared her positive experiences with cannabis through numerous media and medical conferences.

At age 12, Jacqueline began searching for a solution for stuttering, which is one of several potential CP symptoms. She found The Emperor Wears no Clothes and was surprised at the purported medical value of cannabis, as it contradicted what she learned in the infamous anti-drug D.A.R.E. program.

The first time Jacqueline tried cannabis, she immediately realized that for the first time in her life, she was not in pain. Her fingers were less hyperextended, and her arm was less tense. Over time, Jacqueline found cannabis mitigated her speech spasms and muscle spasticity and helps rebuild muscles after working out. In addition, cannabis has anxiolytic and appetite-stimulating properties that benefit her.

In the past, Jacqueline has tried muscle relaxers and the prescription medicine Provigal, but they were largely ineffective or caused significant side effects. She now uses a wide variety of cannabis products, and has tried "smoking joints, smoking bongs, smoking pipes, vaporizing oil, vaporizing herb, vaporizing wax, tinctures, teas, edibles, capsules, eating oil, hash eating, salves, lotions, patches, and dabs." Jacqueline notes that dabs are remarkably effective for immediate pain relief, lasting twice as long as smoked cannabis.

Her specialty, the cannabis "dirty chai", is a mixture of chai tea with ground cannabis, hot water, cream or almond milk (for fat), and espresso. Using a range of medicines allows Jacqueline to most comprehensively address her symptoms.

Jacqueline believes transdermal cannabis patches and topical extracts will most effectively benefit other CP patients. Such medicines can deliver sustained and targeted cannabis doses.

"I would really like to see a cannabis patch made from hemp fabric." – Jacqueline Patterson

Cannabis works best when combined with nutrition, exercise, and meditative practices. This is a truth Jacqueline understands quite well. She has physical therapy and massage sessions and is an avid practitioner of yoga.

She says, "These methods help relax, strengthen, and tone the muscles without a psychoactive high."

Jacqueline believes cannabis and these other practices are true medicines, as they help heal the body, unlike pharmaceuticals which generally mask symptoms and cause debilitating side effects. She is currently active and doing well, always seeking out new ways to improve her health."

Source: https://illegallyhealed.com/relief-from-cerebral-palsy

Case Study #71: Gavin's Remarkable Turnaround From Cerebral Palsy and Autism

"I sensed true desperation almost immediately when Rebecca brought her son Gavin in to see me. The despair was nearly palpable, even in Gavin's two grandmothers who had accompanied them to the office. Gavin himself appeared oblivious to his surroundings, made little to no eye contact and was very hyperactive and distracted, moving around the office the entire time. A cute child wearing a little fedora and glasses, his face showed little affect and we made no connection. "We need help so badly," the small group said to me, "we can no longer live like this."

Rebecca is a stay at home mother with a special education degree whose first child Gavin was born six weeks early. While he had low muscle tone, something you'd expect from a preemie, he also didn't reach his early milestones, and at around age two, Gavin's health and development began to really fall apart.

He was nearly two when he walked and had little to no language at age three. Ultimately diagnosed with complex partial seizures, cerebral palsy and an unknown genetic anomaly, as well as cyclical vomiting and autism, Gavin was prescribed the anticonvulsant Keppra for his seizures. He was three years old, and the effects were immediate. While the seizures stopped, Gavin's autistic behaviors increased, and within two months his meltdowns became uncontrollable. Rebecca and her husband had read about "Keppra rage," a well-documen-ted side effect, but they wanted to control the seizures and were hesitant to take him off of the drug or add another one.

During this time, Rebecca saw the CNN documentary "Weed" and began to explore cannabis as a possible treatment. When she asked Gavin's neurologist about trying cannabis, he ignorantly asked her if she was going to "blow smoke in his face." She was discouraged by this response but kept searching online for information and found support on Facebook. She eventually brought Gavin to my office in early 2014. With his behaviour out of control, life with Gavin had become a daily struggle.

I started Gavin on CBD-rich cannabis oil, given by mouth. The effects were immediate. **Within 10 days, Gavin, previously non-verbal, began speaking.**

The change was so dramatic that Rebecca wanted to try weaning him off the Keppra to see if his seizures might also be controlled. She switched neurologists and found a partner who helped her to wean Gavin off Keppra over five months. When he was completely off the drug, an initial EEG showed some seizure activity, but Rebecca asked for three months to adjust the dosage of CBD before trying other pharmaceuticals. **The subsequent 48-hour EEG showed no seizure activity**, and Gavin hasn't needed any further antiepileptic medications.

Although the use of CBD-rich oil for a number of months resulted in seizure freedom, improved verbal ability and improved behaviour, Gavin continued to have some unwanted behaviours related to his autism. It was at this point that we added THC-rich oil in the mornings and afternoons to help him to be calm and focused. **As we hoped, his behaviour improved significantly.**

Rebecca still marvels at the dramatic turnaround in Gavin due to cannabis medicine. In addition to seizure control, Gavin's incredible improvements in speech and autistic behaviors thrill her the most. Although everyone who knew Gavin saw that he was quite intelligent (even the speech pathologist had given him an iPad with communication apps because they knew his capabilities), he had no real language or any imaginary play.

One afternoon soon after Gavin began taking CBD oil, Rebecca was in her bedroom folding laundry. She looked up to see Gavin walking in with the laundry basket. He placed it on the floor, stepped into it and declared, "Look, Mom! I'm an astronaut!"

Rebecca has had to experiment with the dose and ratio of CBD and THC, and has ultimately found that an overall CBD:THC ratio of 1:1 is giving him the best results.

Despite a relatively high dose of THC, Gavin has no adverse side effects from cannabis use. He does not experience any psychoactivity. He is able to make connections in his kindergarten class, to fit in with his peers and to transition throughout the day with ease. He is happy and thriving, and reports from school are outstanding. The speech pathologist has even taken away the iPad with the communication apps because he doesn't need it anymore!

Gavin is now five years old, and his story moves me as both physician and mother. When Rebecca sent me a video recently of him reciting the Pledge of Allegiance and breaking into "You're a Grand Old Flag," I was moved to tears. Although not every patient has this level of improvement, Gavin's story is an example of why cannabis treatment must be an available option for all children with severe medical conditions. His quality of life has been improved so significantly that he is able to participate in his life fully as all children deserve."

Source: www.marijuana.com/news/2017/04/five-year-old-gavins-cannabis-success-story-will-move-you-to-tears

Case Study #72: Cerebral Palsy Treated With Cannabis Extracts

"My son had seizures a few hours after birth. He was transported to NICU (Newborn Intensive Care Unit) in Nebraska, spent a month there, where he was tested for genetic and metabolic disorders. Multiple brain scans showed severe damage to the whole brain and particularly bad in occipital areas. He was sent home on hospice care and seizure medications, with no plan of treatment or follow up care.

I believe Cannabis saved my son's life. He hasn't had any recurring seizures, no further hospitalizations or illnesses, and is progressing developmentally, though it is a slower pace than a typical child.

He has generally slept well through the night and has learned to use his hands to play with toys, to clap and make word sounds, to laugh and express his emotions.

[We give him] high THC glycerin-based tincture made from a Sativa strain. The tincture is given three times per day, orally. I feel that my decision was the right one and the only one, and that I was able to help my child when the medical 'professionals' were not.

I read research articles on Google scholar, pertaining to testing on animals that had experienced neonatal encephalopathy and oxygen deprivation at birth. I was part of multiple support groups on Facebook that offered parent information and support. I follow other journeys on Facebook and I constantly read new research and information articles online on this topic.

I used to use Cannabis recreationally and was slightly familiar with different options and strains, but since my son was sick we have learned much more about the process of growing plants and the different benefits of Cannabis for treating various ailments and conditions."

Source: www.cannabisoilsuccessstories.com/cerebral-palsy.html

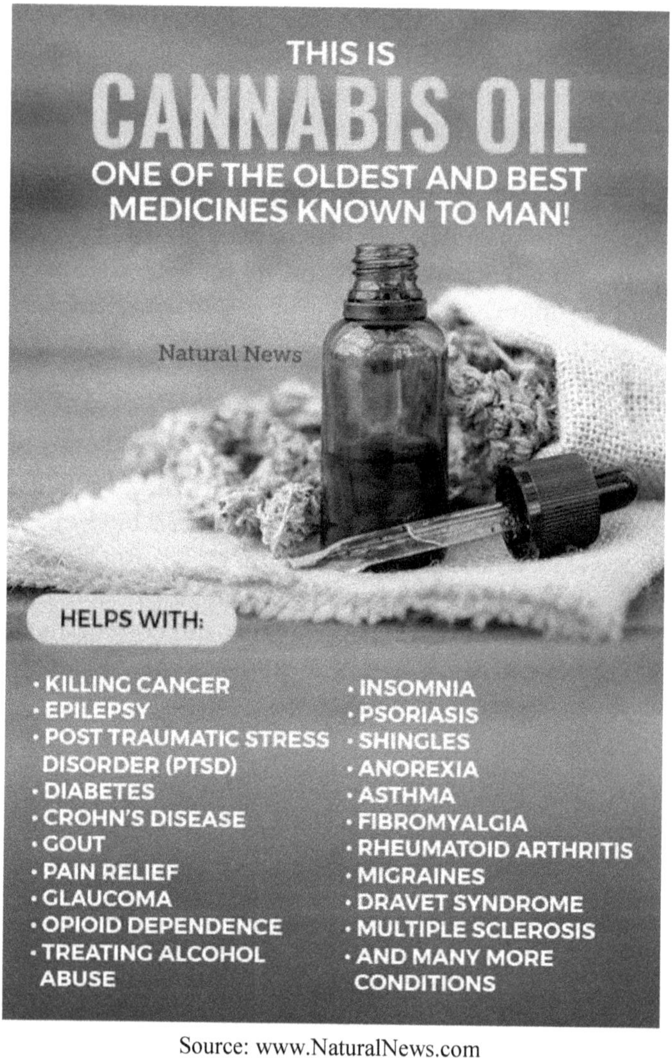

Source: www.NaturalNews.com

CHAPTER 17

Multiple Sclerosis and Cannabis

Multiple Sclerosis is the condition which has most commonly been associated with the therapeutic use of cannabis. It was the increasing illicit use of cannabis to treat MS that led to the House of Lords Science and Technology Committee inquiry in 1998, in the UK. The approval of Sativex (nabiximols) for the treatment of spasticity in MS is the first licensed cannabis medicine in modern times.

There is a clear consensus amongst scientists and doctors that cannabis is safe and effective as a palliative treatment for MS. Further promising research is underway into whether cannabinoids may have a curative effect by promoting repair of the myelin sheath.

Case Study #73: Upper Body Use Regained And Able To Walk Instantly Thanks to Cannabis Oil

"I have been a section 56 Cannabis member for 25 years. **I regained motor skills in my legs instantly and was able to walk again upon smoking my first joint.** I regained my upper body usage and returned to work as an auto mechanic for another 23 years, I feel, due to the use of Cannabis.

155

I infuse coconut oil and Cannabis and ingest it as well as use it topically. I use alcohol-extracted Cannabis Oil I vaporize as well as smoke my Cannabis. I do not have a set dosing schedule, I just took Cannabis at times I felt my body was in need.

My father passed away from Multiple Sclerosis at the age of 45 after spending the final 10 years in a hospital bed. I was diagnosed at the age of 23 with the same symptoms as my father except he lost his sight, I did not. **I feel Cannabis is the reason that I have lived a longer, more productive life than he did.** Cannabis is a medicine that saved me and I can only hope it can do the same for others."

Source: www.cannabisoilsuccessstories.com/multiple-sclerosis-ii.html

Case Study #74: Cannabis Oil Changed My Life

"[Before Cannabis extract]: The onset of MS included being bedridden, having dizziness, nausea, extreme vertigo, vomiting and developing optic neuritis which left me blind in my right eye.

[After taking Cannabis extract]: Life is normal, I function well; **it has changed my life.** I ingest Cannabis in my smoothie. I vaporize Cannabis. I take Cannabis coconut oil extract, and I take straight Cannabis Oil; the Oil has been mostly Indica strains, high in THC.

Dosing Regime:
- Five grams of decarboxylated Cannabis a day
- Two mil of coconut oil-Cannabis Oil extract
- One rice-sized dose of concentrated Cannabis Oil daily

I feel fabulous about my health. I am healthy because of Cannabis and a healthy diet and I know Cannabis has changed my life and helped me to stay healthy."

Source: www.cannabisoilsuccessstories.com/multiple-sclerosis--female-ontario.html

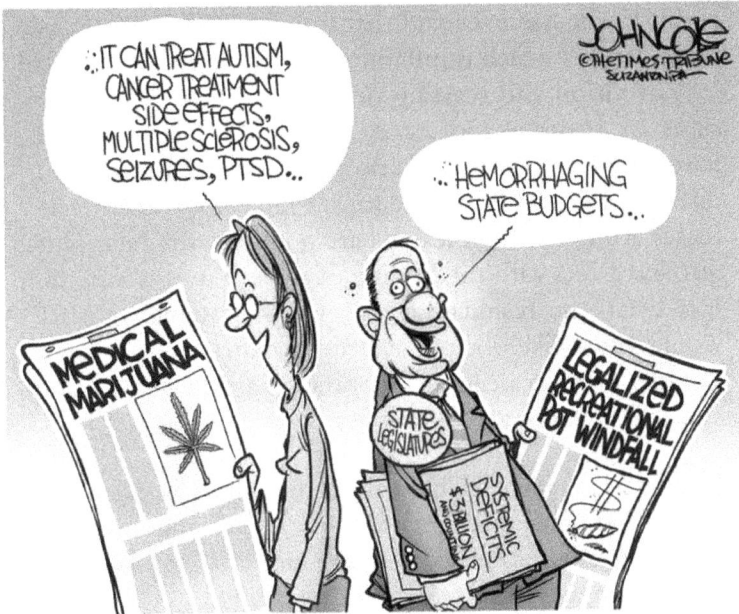

Case Study #75: My MS Specialist Told Me "You No Longer Need To Come In For Follow Ups!"

"I had constant neurological symptoms for eight years with 30 brain and spine lesions. I had no quality of life and could barely get out of bed, with crushing fatigue. I was losing my eyesight and the ability walk.

I am now a healthier and happier version of the girl who got sick 13 years ago. I can climb mountains again. This year I graduated as a Nutritional Therapy Practitioner. **My life is a miracle! Cannabis Oil was huge in my recovery**, but I do not believe I would be where I was today if it was not for diet and detoxification. I follow the Wahls protocol, which is a nutrient-rich paleo diet. I do best on Wahls' level 3, which is a ketogenic diet.

My Multiple Sclerosis [MS] specialist told me at my last appointment that I no longer need to come in for follow ups. She let me know I am the first person with MS she has ever said that too. I had many cases of optic neuritis which is inflammation in the eye leading to loss of vision and scarring on the eye nerve. I have no signs of scarring and 20/20 vision. My doctor could hardly believe that there is no damage left after over 20 different cases of Optic Neuritis. I have not had an MRI to see if my 30 brain lesions are gone but my Neurologist and I feel with the healing of my eye nerves and the fact I have no residual neurological symptoms, an MRI would most likely show no more damage. Emotional healing has also been an important part of my journey and that includes avoiding stress.

I use a Cannabis Oil high in THC, which is extracted with food-grade alcohol. I took a 300 mg dose of Cannabis Oil before bed. During the day I smoked and vaped for relief from the symptoms.

When I started Cannabis Oil I thought it was just for symptoms and to help me get off all the prescription medications I was on. The more I learn the more I believe **it helped heal my brain and put my Lyme disease in remission.** I believe it put my body into homeostasis, allowing me to heal."

Source: www.cannabisoilsuccessstories.com/lyme-disease--40-yr-old-female.html

CHAPTER 18

Lyme Disease and Cannabis

Lyme disease is known as the great imitator since is mimics so many other diseases. It's for this reason that it can be incredibly difficult to diagnose and treat in time. In this chapter, I share three case studies of inspiring individuals who treated their Lyme disease using cannabis oil and the results they each found.

Case Study #76: Out of a Wheelchair and Walking Again Thanks to Cannabis

"I was treated for Lyme Disease conventionally and non-conventionally for seven years with zero improvement (I was also living in a mould environment for more than seven years unbeknownst to me). I was in a wheelchair after year five of treatment for Lyme and other conditions. I couldn't leave my home for more than a doctor appointment and was mostly confined to my bed. My memory was non-existent.

Medications prescribed: Ativan 3mg a day, Beta blockers and two pain killers, Doxycycline, Rifampin, Zoloft.

After experimenting for seven years with Cannabis and homeopathics and addressing methylation (with corrective supplements and homeopathics), I'm out of a wheelchair and out running errands for myself as well as helping heal others. Zero depression. Zero panic attacks. Pain completely gone. Vision has improved tenfold as well as my hearing. Life is now looking amazing to me and I'm filled with hope for a full recovery. My brain is now sharp as a tack. It took a full approach of supplements as well as my own remedy creation of THCa, low THC and only CBDa at night. Straight CBD gave me massive anxiety as my immune system was in full TH2 cycle.

I used THCa, low THC and CBDa in my own recipe I create. I've not had it lab tested for potency or Cannabis compounds. I just continued to experiment and keep track with 72 journals. I used my immune status as a guide via lab work.

I feel amazing with my choice to use cannabis as an adjunct therapy with other supplants for methylation, clean Paleo diet and energy work. **My life is incredibly different now and I'm so grateful for our medicine!"**

Source: www.cannabisoilsuccessstories.com/lyme-disease-and-co-infections.html

Case Study #77: Beth Schultz treated Lyme Disease Naturally

"I have a diagnosis of MS. I also test positive for Lyme disease. I had over 30 brain and spine lesions that look exactly like MS. I treated with antibiotics for 8 years and still had symptoms. I finally started to treat all naturally 4 years ago and **have been in remission for 3 years.** I think diet is the most important thing for both diseases.

I follow the Wahls protocol and it has given me back life. I also take a big dose of cannabis oil before bed. My cannabis oil is high in THC and has some CBD. Please

Google Dr. Wahls Ted Talk and learn about her miraculous recovery using a Paleo diet for her PPMS."

Source: www.medicaljane.com/2015/05/22/doctor-believes-cannabidiol-paste-could-be-a-potential-cure-for-lyme-disease/

Case Study #78: Lyme Disease Cured Thanks to Cannabis Extracts

"The beginning of my journey with Lyme disease is similar to most. My ending, however, is playing out quite differently than most. I found a tick behind my ear at the age of fourteen and had various health problems for seven years before I was finally diagnosed with Lyme disease, Lupus, Mycoplasma, Bartonella, and Babesia. After two years my Lupus, Mycoplasma, Bartonella and Babesia are entirely eradicated. As far as my Lyme disease goes, **I now have zero symptoms.** My remaining ones are a result of withdrawals from the prescriptions I so naively started taking when I was initially diagnosed.

How am I already returning to a healthy lifestyle only two years after forgetting to read, write, walk and talk? Well, a wealth of credit is owed to the Buhner protocol. I would not be where I am today without it. Still, I had one last giant "hump" in healing to get over after a year on the protocol. So I took a shot in the dark which, for me, turned out to be the path to light. **I decided to make my own cannabis oil** and began taking it every waking hour.

I now owe my life to this fascinating herb and am hopeful some of you will find strength and encouragement through this information.

For a year and a half I had over ten seizures a day. I tried every treatment I could find, exhausting outlets in both conventional and holistic medicine. Desperately searching for answers, **I stumbled across what turned out to be one of the most profound facts I have ever learned.**

Marijuana contains one of the most potent anticonvulsants in the world. Controversy over the subject was meaningless at that point, as the herb offered a possible solution to one of my most debilitating symptoms. As it turned out, **smoking marijuana not only controlled my seizures, it completely cured them.**

With that in mind, I moved forward with my research. If it could do for seizures what no other plant or prescription could do, what could it do for Lyme? What I found was nothing short of fascinating, and essentially lifesaving.

Cannabis has over 700 healing components. [...] I began using a vaporizer to get more cannabinoids. My rate of improvement significantly sped up when I did this. Naturally, this motivated me to take treatment one step further and find out what the results of taking cannabis oil would do for me. **After only a month of taking it I was able to return to work and school and began to drive and have a social life again.** Now, I am finally planning to move out and be independent for the first time in years. Basically, I am returning to a lifestyle that I was once unsure I would ever see again thanks to the immense healing power of cannabis oil."

Source: www.collective-evolution.com/2013/09/12/amazing-story-the-healing-power-of-cannabis-oil-on-lyme-disease-and-lyme-co-infections/

CHAPTER 19

Inflammation, Chronic Pain, Fibromyalgia and Lupus

The mainstream medical solution for pain is usually to administer strong—and sometimes deadly—painkillers. However, in this chapter I share six testimonials of people who have cured their chronic pain, inflammation, Fibromyalgia, Lupus and other related issues, simply by using cannabis oil.

A study revealed that **medical cannabis use effectively eases inflammation, swelling, tension, and sore muscles.** A team of Canadian health experts have examined 215 adult chronic pain patients as part of the study. The patients were given flowers, concentrates, or edible cannabis during the study's duration. The results were then compared with a control cohort of 216 healthy patients.

Patients who took medicinal cannabis exhibited significant declines in pain and increased quality of life, the researchers reported. Likewise, patients in the cannabis group attained mark reductions in anxiety, depression, and fatigue.

Let us explore how cannabis can help people suffering from chronic pain, as illustrated by the following six case studies.

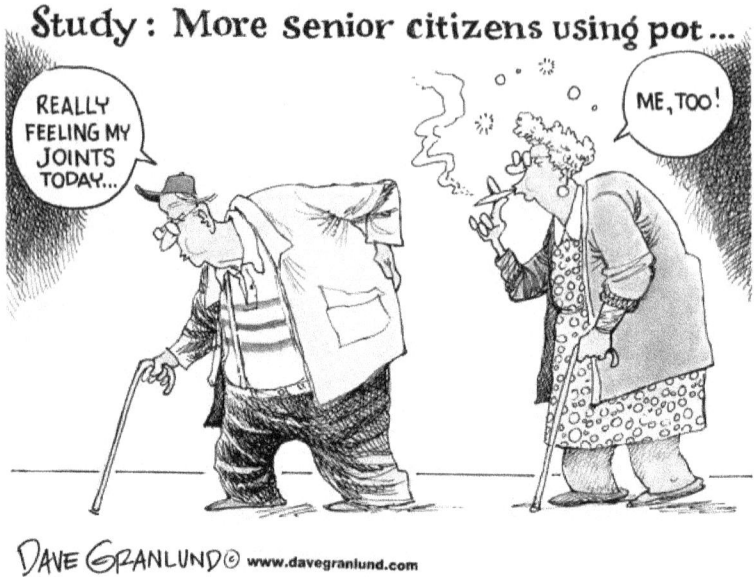

Study: More senior citizens using pot...

REALLY FEELING MY JOINTS TODAY...

ME, TOO!

DAVE GRANLUND© www.davegranlund.com

Case Study #79: Extreme Pain Due To Chronic Inflammation of the Spine, Healed With Cannabis

"I have a primary immune impairment since childhood. That means basically that one is born with an HIV/AIDS-like immunodeficiency, but it's not caused by a virus and it's not contagious, but a genetic "disorder". This I've had now already since birth. But due to various circumstances, and a healthcare that is beneath all contempt, I have remained undiagnosed until recently.

I've never received adequate care or treatment in Sweden. Instead of examining me, they have chosen to drug me. So now the disease progression has led to a near critical point, when all my symptoms rapidly have become aggravated. I've gone in and out of the emergency rooms the recent weeks.

My chronic symptoms are, among other things; **extreme pain due to chronic inflammation of the spine**, which caused the bone changes and a narrowing of the spinal cord, which gives constant nerve aches in the body, and intense spasticity, cramps and nerves impacts, chronic nausea and 2.5 years of daily vomiting.

This, the Swedish healthcare has medicated with various drugs on prescription. I've received prescription tramadol, buprenorphine, oxycontin (synthetic heroin), Valium, Ritalin (amphetamine-like substance), Zolpidem/Stilnoct, Lyrica, flunitranzepam and a number of other hard drugs, quite legally, paid for by taxpayers, to pick up free at the pharmacy.

My symptoms require a number of narcotics on prescription, if I want to be treated with legal substances. But after the first time I've had experienced opioid withdrawal, because of physical dependence on tramadol, which the doctors said was just a "little stronger painkiller," I started researching on alternative ways to get relief for my symptoms. I'm involved in several international support groups for chronically ill people, and in all of them, **medical marijuana is praised as a miracle cure for people who suffer daily**, from various chronic diseases, just like me. I've smoked cannabis in Finland as a young teenager, since it was decriminalized there. Many seniors with rheumatism had one or two plants in the window, it wasn't uncommon at all. And even today you can legally collect cannabis in the Finnish pharmacies on prescription.

I decided to try it for medicinal purposes, if it might give me even a little relief of some of the symptoms. As well as having a chronical fatigue that cannot be described, partly because of the body's impaired immune system, and because it was often impossible to sleep due to the constant nerve aches. So, I figured it was worth the risk, even though it's illegal in Sweden.

165

My friends came over and brought some cannabis with them. **The first time I smoked for medical reasons, after several years of total abstinence from all drugs (except those on the prescription), I started to cry. The feeling is indescribable. All my symptoms disappeared, as if by magic.** It took only 2-3 puffs of a joint, and my symptoms disappeared almost immediately. I had no pain ANYWHERE in my body! And no nausea! And not much later I even had an appetite to eat without nauseating! A feeling I had not experienced in a very, very long time.

The feeling was so incredible, I had forgotten what a pain-free state feels like, I was so used to the pain. [...] Since cannabis is proven in a number of international researches, to be, among other things; antibacterial, immune-regulating/enhancing, anti-inflammatory, analgesic, neuron-repairing, anticonvulsant, and possibly even cancer-killing. And with no proven, adverse side effects, and no risk of overdose, the opposite to all prescription drugs I've received, where the risk of death from overdose are very high. So, the decision was easy.

If you had seen my little son's suffering before, when he tried to comfort his ailing mother, who spent 80-90% of the time in bed, in a half-conscious state, your hearts would burst. I was often too tired to even smile at my son. I had to whisper in his ear, "I smile in my heart, but can't manage to show it now ..." I raised my son all by myself, without any support from his father, for 10 years. He's the most tragic victim of this disease drama.

Today he's a happy guy, because he has an energetic and healthier mom."

Source: https://illegallyhealed.com/my-body-my-illness-my-choice

Case Study #80: 42 Year Old Christine Stenquist
Gets Her Life Back Thanks To Cannabis

"Christine Stenquist is a 42-year-old mother of four from Kaysville, Utah, who says using medical cannabis gave her life back and that more patients, even in states where it is illegal, need to make themselves heard.

Christine spent two decades in excruciating pain, cycling through pain meds, trapped in the quiet darkness of her bedroom. In 2012 she tried medical cannabis and since that time has weaned off her pharmaceuticals and founded the Drug Policy Project of Utah. By coming out of the cannabis closet, she has led the charge for medical cannabis legislation in the state.

Christine was raised in Miami by her father, a proud Vietnam Veteran and well-respected narcotics officer. Christine's father participated in the second-biggest cocaine bust in Miami history and served on the force for 27 years, and it wasn't until she received his blessing that she tried cannabis.

Christine has been suffering from severe and chronic migraines since the age of seven. **In her twenties a tumour was discovered in her brain** and in 1996 she was diagnosed with an acoustic neuroma and underwent brain surgery to remove a portion of the tumour. Doctors could not remove the entire tumour for fear of causing nerve damage to her face and body. The tumour is benign and portions of it still sit on various nerves in her brain.

The **symptoms of fibromyalgia** came 15 months after brain surgery. She started having muscle spasms, vertigo, balance issues and unrelenting migraine pain. As her symptoms became increasingly severe, she could no longer hold a job, and so began over a decade in pain cycling through prescription drugs.

Her doctors continued to prescribe various painkillers, steroids, anti-depressants and anti-seizure medications. She received a steady dose of morphine through fentanyl patches and 450mg fentanyl suckers for breakthrough pain. She was prescribed over 60 Percocet a month, received trigger point injections at a pain clinic and got nerve ablations, to no avail.

Christine cycled through over 30 drugs. She was she comfortable being so heavily medicated. But, she says, it was all her doctors could do to treat the blinding pain.

In the fall of 2011 Christine became so ill she lost most of her mental and physical function. After three to five weeks in bed she was no longer walking or eating and wasting quickly. She was suffering painful migraines that kept her awake vomiting from the pain and has started having seizures. At that point her husband had to physically carry her into the shower just to bathe.

Christine says the low point came that winter when she had been in so much pain that she cut her arms to see if she could feel it anymore. Her husband got nervous and took her to the hospital where a doctor asked her if she was suicidal. She said that she wasn't, but she was just in too much pain. The doctor offered her more medication.

"I had been on that stuff for years, I couldn't do it anymore. **My husband collapsed on the ground, he was just sobbing** because after three months of me in bed and him caring for me and still maintaining a full-time job and caring for our children, it had just become too much." says Christine. "We had hit the point where there were no more answers, no more help, no relief."

In 2013, the accepted success of medical cannabis started to work its way into the mainstream via Dr. Sanjay Gupta, CNN's chief medical correspondent. **Christine began to wonder if medical cannabis could help her,** but it wasn't until her father, the former narcotics cop, suggested she try it that she finally decided to do it.

"I am feeling good," she says. As time passed Christine weaned herself off more pharmaceuticals and today is **pharmaceutical free and can walk, drive and be present in her family's lives.** After regaining her health, Christine founded the Drug Policy Project of Utah and became the executive director of the organization."

Source: https://illegallyhealed.com/finding-relief/

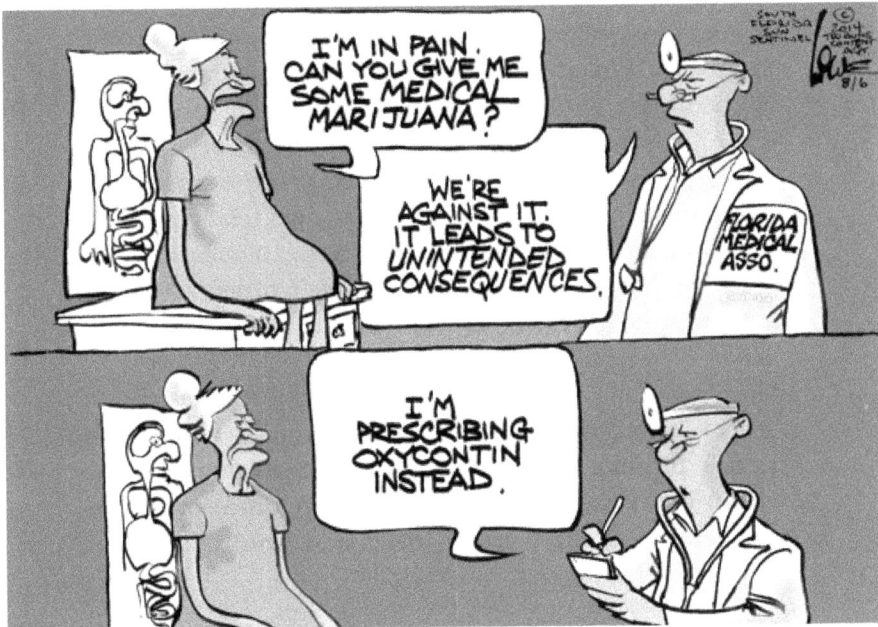

Case Study #81: My Girls Have Their Mom Back
After 10 Year Battle With Chronic Pain and Opiate Addiction

"After a horrific near-death car accident in October 2006, I was on opiates and pharmaceuticals for over 10 years. I went through 15 surgeries in 10 years and that's a hard thing to do without pain pills. I did not smoke weed, drink, party, none of it growing up. Before my accident I went to school, got my degree, married, had children, a career; I was a "soccer mom" who believed Cannabis was the Devil's Lettuce.

Unfortunately, these medications destroyed my body and have left me with a mind that I struggle with every second of the day. While on pharmaceuticals I was stuck away in my bedroom for years, bloated, tired, sluggish, foggy headed, confused, obese at 410lbs, out of shape, horrible health, Type 2 diabetes, not involved in my family's life, lost all my friends but a very few, my own relatives called me a drug addict and distanced from me. It was an awful existence, but what's so scary is I didn't realize just how bad it was, until I came out of my opiate fog last year.

After beginning to smoke a little Cannabis in October of 2014, I started noticing a bit of improvement. **Next, we tried a topical; wow, what relief for my nerve pain, within just minutes.** We knew we were onto something and decided to start having me ingest Cannabis Oil in May of 2015.

After only two months I was able to get off the 1,500mg of Metformin; my diabetes was gone (I'm supposed to say 'in remission'), and **within only three months I was off all opiates** (including Oxycontin, Percocet and nerve medication Gabapentin). **I was working again within only three months, and I had not worked in 15 years!** I dropped 100lbs in less than a year from Cannabis and plant healing; a total loss so far of 193lbs.

Now I'm sleeping for 4-5 hours at a time; it used to be 2-3 hours. I'm treating my conditions every day, all day, with Cannabis. **I'm out and about living and thriving now because of Cannabis.** My youngest daughter recently said, "Mom, you're a much better mom on Cannabis than you ever were on pills." Right there is how I know it was all worth it. My girls have their mom again, my family has me back and I can now share my healing story with others, so they learn there's an alternative to pharmaceuticals.

I now ingest Cannabis Oil capsules, eat edibles, use topicals and smoke on a daily basis. I have asthma, so I try to vape since it's easier on my lungs. I have kept a pain and cannabis journal from the beginning, which has helped me IMMENSELY when figuring out what has worked or how I need to change things up a bit, my body is still healing and will for years. The very best way I can describe **what cannabis did was bring homeostasis to my body**. One by one the meds and supplements fell away, week by week.

I use cannabis on a daily basis throughout my day. Currently I make Cannabis Oil capsules weekly, apply topicals multiple times a day and I eat edibles as needed for breakthrough pain; just as I used a Percocet before. I also smoke off and on as needed to keep my pain, anxiety, PTSD, facial tic, shoulder tic and PAWS quieted. I have learned to make my own infused coconut oil to add in my food and make edibles with. I am constantly trying different strains to see what will work best. My tics are made worse by some terpenes, which is another reason for the pain journal; I can tailor make my medicine just for me.

I began getting cannabis oil in May 2015 by ingesting a half grain of rice size with a spoonful of peanut butter. After three months of this micro-dosing, **we learned the body absorbs the Cannabis Oil better if it's mixed**

with a carrier oil. We began making capsules mixed with flaxseed oil. We learned that the flaxseed binds with the Cannabis Oil and made it water soluble. We continued this for about six months until my body healed even further and changed a bit. The further along I get from detoxing, the more conditions pop up; things left from years of pharmaceuticals in my body. At my highest during immediate detox I got up to ingesting 3 grams of oil a day. We believe that could have been less if we had originally been informed to mix with a carrier oil, so the uptake is better through the blood barrier in the liver. I'm 14 months clean from opiates now and am ingesting approximately one gram of oil a day in capsule form, eating four edible cookies a day, smoke about three times a day and still use my topicals regularly."

[...] "We tried a topical [our friends] suggested, and the quick results were amazing. Within a few minutes I could feel the blood circulating and my arm and hand getting warm. **And, within about 10 minutes, I was starting to have relief for the pins, needles, itching and burning nerve pain I have constantly.** From there we started ingesting cannabis oil and eventually started learning how to make my own medicine.

Cannabis has given me my life back; my girls have their mom and my family and friends can't believe the shocking difference in just months. My life has changed 180 degrees in just the last year. I sleep at least half the night now, which is a huge improvement; I'm out of the house socializing and am able to be a cannabis activist now, sharing my story on a daily basis."

Source: www.cannabisoilsuccessstories.com/chronic-regional-pain-syndrome-- crps-.html

Case Study #82: Mandy Declined Surgery to Fight Painful Hidradenitis Suppurativa With Cannabis Oil

"It is remarkable how many conditions cannabis is able to alleviate. From common diseases to rare conditions that most people have never heard of, many patients attest to the widespread effectiveness of cannabis medicine.

Mandy began experiencing the symptoms of hidradenitis suppurativa (HS) during her pregnancy in 2006. In this condition, painful, inflamed red nodules appear in various places across the body. For Mandy, these first appeared in her groin area. Doctors initially wrote off the inflammation as ingrown hairs or hormonal changes.

After giving birth, the sores got worse instead of getting better. She was eventually diagnosed by her family physician with Stage 1 HS. Given the early stage of the disease and other personal reasons, Mandy did not receive any medication at the time.

In 2010, her condition worsened causing significant pain, infectious issues, and bleeding concerns. From this point and for the next two years, Mandy tried numerous medications and surgery, all of which failed to stop the disease from progressing to Stage 3 by 2012.

She even had to leave her much-loved position in histopathology at the local hospital due to complications.

In August 2013, Mandy had numerous intravenous clindamycin treatments, along with an oral course of the antibiotic drug. It helped with the inflammation but did little for the pain. Unfortunately, this treatment apparently led to an infection.

Mandy was referred to a surgeon in November 2013 and was told invasive surgery would be needed to stop the HS, as it has now deeply penetrated the skin. She declined the surgery due to the risks. Prior to this, Mandy had done some research on the potential of cannabis to treat her condition and had also been smoking it to treat pain.

It was not until she learned of Corrie Yelland, who beat terminal anal canal cancer with cannabis oil, that Mandy became determined to undergo cannabis extract therapy. She received a cannabis recommendation from her doctor and began treatment in April 2014. Mandy decided that she should attack her disease full force and attempt the "60 grams in 90 days" treatment. She also used cannabis oil topically on her HS wounds to heal the condition as completely as possible.

Mandy started with small doses and increased as fast as she could tolerate. The medicine made her very tired, but also instantly relieved her pain. **Within five months, all the HS related wounds had nearly disappeared, and Mandy also lost 50 pounds. She finally felt liberated and free.**

Full strength cannabis oils have been most effective for Mandy's symptoms. She tried tinctures made with a sunflower oil or alcohol base, but they were not strong enough to prevent flare-ups. However, those she has had since her initial treatment have never been as strong as before.

The original oil that worked best was made with the strain Banana Kush. As a maintenance dose, she takes 2 drops of oil 2-3 times daily. She puts the drops on parchment paper and freezes them, then swallows them like small pills. While Mandy has never weighed her doses, starting small and slowly working to higher levels has been very effective for her.

A 2013 study found that topically applied THC could attenuate allergic inflammation, which the researchers determined had "implications for the future development of strategies to harness cannabinoids for the treatment of inflammatory skin diseases." An earlier study found cannabinoids may benefit psoriasis, which shares some similarities with HS.

Mandy states: "When I was suffering of large wounds I applied cannabis oil directly into the holes and watched it melt into the tunnel. A couple of weeks later and the tunnel had healed to the surface. **Cannabis oil has given me my life back. I no longer dread waking up every morning.** It is not agonizing to walk or wear clothes. I finally feel I am at peace with myself."

Source: https://illegallyhealed.com/declining-skin-surgery-to-try-cannabis-oil

Case Study #83: Ginamarie Pezzi Takes Back Control From Chronic Illnesses Thanks to Cannabis

"Ginamarie Pezzi has been through a lot in her life. From a young age, she suffered from abuse and trauma that created and exacerbated health conditions, including insomnia, fibromyalgia, morbid obesity, sciatica, osteo-arthritis, PTSD, and Type 2 diabetes.

For decades, Ginamarie fought debilitating conditions with surgery and pharmaceuticals. At one point, her daily pain averaged between 6 and 9 (out of 10). She was taking 240mg of methadone every day along with eight other pharmaceuticals. These prescriptions did little to help and actually caused damage.

In May 2000, Ginamarie had a successful stomach bypass surgery, which helped her lose 200 pounds. While this helped in the short term, it ultimately contributed to long-term nutritional deficiencies. The PTSD, fibromyalgia, and insomnia also created a cycle that mutually worsened each condition's symptoms.

In early 2013, Ginamarie finally decided to change her approach. She stopped using pharmaceuticals and applied for an Oregon Medical Marijuana Program (OMMP) card as a last resort to restore her health. After being approved, she acquired 7 grams of a high-THC cannabis strain and vaporized it with a VaporGenie.

Ginamarie says that **after only three hits had a remarkable healing effect. Her pain dropped by two levels almost immediately** and she could breathe better. Most incredibly, that night she had the best night of sleep of her life. "Three hits is all it took and I could feel the medicine working right away."

Since her first cannabis experience, Ginamarie has been steadily improving. She ingests edibles, cannabis oil, and cannabis tincture when possible. Some setbacks have inhibited Ginamarie's progress, such as moving to Las Vegas and losing steady access to cannabis. However, she will soon have a large yield from her legal grow, which will enable her to consume cannabis in several forms.

"Cannabis allows me to heal and continue functioning, but you have to maintain treatment," said Ginamarie."

Source: https://illegallyhealed.com/cannabis-for-insomnia-ginamarie-says-yes

Case Study #84: Kristen Kourtney Recovers From Rheumatoid Arthritis and Lupus By Juicing Cannabis

"Most people associate cannabis extract medicine with solvent-derived cannabis oils, which are further broken down into high-THC and high-CBD oils. There has been a growing movement to juice cannabis, a method that preserves raw acidic cannabinoids. When heated, THCA and CBDA decarboxylate to THC and CBD, which have different properties. Heat can also destroy valuable terpenoids that have been proven to work synergistically with cannabinoids. With juice, all of these compounds are preserved.

Dr. William Courtney in California has pioneered the field of juiced cannabis. His experience, along with his wife Kristen, was detailed in the 2011 documentary 'Leaf'.

Since the age of 16, Kristen battled rheumatoid arthritis and lupus, which resulted in her being bedridden for four years. Doctors said she wouldn't make it to 30 and would never have children.

Kristen began juicing cannabis, which led to her relatively quick recovery. She now has three children, and when juicing displays virtually no symptoms of her previously debilitating diseases."

Source: https://illegallyhealed.com/juicing-cannabis

CHAPTER 20

Healing From Crohn's Disease, Colitis, and Digestive Issues

Can cannabis oil and extracts be beneficial for those suffering with Crohn's, Colitis, and other digestive issues? In this chapter I share with you five incredible stories of people who believe it can.

Case Study #85: This is How I'm Conquering Crohn's Naturally

"In the past, I have had trouble talking about having Crohn's Disease. It was just a reality I have lived with for over a decade but one I was loathed to discuss. The subject is emotionally difficult to explain because it is personal and unpleasant.

I felt compelled to share my story a couple years ago, as I weaned off the only pharmaceutical drug I was taking, Remicade, and have embarked on **the journey of conquering my Crohn's naturally through cannabis, diet and lifestyle.** Since that time, I have had the pleasure of meeting hundreds of people around the world

179

embarking on the same healing journey. We are learning and healing together.

Studies have proven that cannabis has a higher success rate than any pharmaceutical drug used to treat Crohn's Disease, without unpleasant or deadly side effects.

My mom was adopted in the 1960s, when laws pertaining to adoption allowed all records, including medical, to remain locked—even fifty years after the laws have changed. Some digging produced some vague birth records showing a great-grandmother and some biological relatives who died of their colon exploding inside of them. My doctors urged me to find family members who had the illness so they could try to find patterns. We found my biological grandmother in Penn-sylvania, but she wanted nothing to do with either me or my family and refused to provide any medical records.

I began fasting in middle school, but I didn't start seriously starving myself to the point of illness until my sophomore year of high school. By my senior year I was in such terrible pain I would double over crying at night, unable to sleep. A nutritionist my doctor sent me to said it was my vegetarian diet and I needed more protein. I started puking everything I ate. The starving became involuntary.

The day I graduated high school all the other students were lined up ready to process into the auditorium discussing their college plans, I was sitting against a wall trying to regain my composure to get up and walk across the stage with everyone else, biting on my hand to get through the pain so hard I broke skin. That summer before college was pretty miserable. I was in and out of doctors' offices while trying to make plans to move 300 miles away for college.

I was diagnosed with Crohn's three days before I moved into the dorms at San Francisco State University. I spent much of my first semester in my dorm bed under mounds of blankets with the heat blasting because I couldn't eat food and I just never could get warm. As it turned out, I had a blockage in my large intestine that had caused inflammation, which in turn shut my whole body down.

[...] We agreed to do the surgery over my spring break in March 2005. Because I was only 18-years-old they wanted to do what they could to not to scar up my body too much, so they did the surgery laparoscopically (with lasers) and pulled the damaged part of my intestine out through my belly button and glued it back together.

I came out of the surgery a little angry. I was even angrier when they started telling me about all the meds they wanted to give me and when they told me that I had an 80 percent chance of having to do this again in two years, and AGAIN two years after that until I would eventually have to carry a colostomy bag because I didn't have enough intestine left. I wasn't going to accept it. The doctors painted a very bleak and expensive picture of my future, right when it was just getting started.

Moving to San Francisco and seeing the dispensary and medical card ads in the back of the free weeklies was a revelation. I was nervous about getting a medical cannabis recommendation... but I knew I didn't want to take any more of those pills, the effects of the pills were worse than the actual Crohn's both mentally and physically.

My first 'pot doctor' put me at ease immediately. Oddly enough **he was the first doctor to ever even ask me about my diet and lifestyle**; my gastroenterologists just wanted to talk about symptoms and drugs. **He started telling me how I should use it for my Crohn's Disease, how it would help me stop the pills and actually feel better.**

Over the years I researched holistic medicine and integrated that into my daily routine. **For the last two** years I have been **100 percent pharmaceutical free, regularly hiking and doing yoga, and eating a whole foods anti-inflammatory diet.**

This March marked 10 years since my surgery and this August will mark 11 since my diagnosis. **I show no signs of needing surgery again.** I have been able to finish an undergraduate degree in 3.5 years (just shy of my goal of three), get a master's, travel, have a career and be an active participant in my life. **My health is one hundred percent attributable to my decision to ignore everyone's discouragement years ago and replace all those drugs with cannabis.**

Cannabis isn't a deadly drug, it is a plant with the potential to replace thousands (if not more) of deadly pharmaceuticals. It's how people like me get to live a quality life. After all, isn't that what we all want?"

Source: https://illegallyhealed.com/conquering-crohns-naturally

Case Study #86: BJ Battles Chronic Digestive Illness With Cannabis

"For most of his life, B.J. has battled a chronic digestive illness. Different doctors have given various diagnoses, including gastritis, irritable bowel syndrome, leaky gut, or other possibilities. The effects of this disease have significantly inhibited B.J.'s ability to lead a normal life.

In addition to perpetual symptoms like nausea, headaches, intestinal issues, and digestive problems, which are common in inflammatory digestive conditions, headaches and joint pain also burdened him. Just eating is a chore, and he usually can only consume certain foods that do not exacerbate symptoms.

B.J. has tried a multitude of pharmaceuticals, including hydrocodone, oxycodone, hyocyamine sulfate, amitriptyline, donnatal, and several others, but none of them did anything to help his condition. In fact, they worsened his quality of life by adding side effects to the litany of things he already had to deal with.

Cannabis is the only medicine that has relieved his symptoms. **According to B.J., smoking or vaporizing cannabis works almost immediately for nausea relief, and the benefits are maintained for hours.** Three or four sessions of cannabis use per day is often enough to deal with the pain, nausea, and digestive issues.

In addition to regaining his appetite, the cannabis actually seems to enhance digestion. Essentially, when eating a certain quantity of food, he will gain more weight when he smokes cannabis than when not.

B.J. says that consuming cannabis edibles has been more useful for improving sleep and reducing pain more so than treating anxiety and nausea.

Research has shown cannabis may inhibit gastric and intestinal motility through activation of CB1 receptors, which allows food to remain in the digestive system longer and thus become better absorbed. B.J. has also experienced relaxed muscles and reduced nightmares during sleep with cannabis.

B.J. says the side effects from cannabis have mostly been positive, such as laughing, talking, and eating more. However, using the wrong strain at the wrong time of day can induce fatigue or demotivation. The wrong dose can also induce anxiety. By carefully tracking his personal responses to different strains and doses, B.J. avoids these symptoms while maximizing therapeutic effects.

B.J. has found that sativa-dominant strains like Durban Poison and Skunk #1 are best for the day, and heavier hybrids or indicas like Northern Lights and Kush are best for the evening. He tailors each bowl to meet his needs at the time.

Although B.J. has reported experiencing significant symptomatic relief from smoking, he still struggles with the disease and believes his overall health is declining. His goal is to move to Colorado, where he could access the concentrated cannabis oil that he believes may actually heal the root causes of his condition.

Given the incredible anecdotal and clinical evidence of cannabis being able to fight inflammatory intestinal conditions like Crohn's disease, it is likely that full extract cannabis oil or juicing raw cannabis would indeed benefit B.J. even more than smoking."

Source: https://illegallyhealed.com/pills-to-cannabis-combating-chronic-illness

Case Study #87: Justine Meader Juices Cannabis To Beat Crohn's Disease

"Justine Meader intimately understands how devastating Crohn's disease can be. As a chronic inflammatory condition of the gastrointestinal tract, Crohn's disease often results in a host of debilitating symptoms including abdominal cramps, malabsorption of nutrients, fatigue, and bowel problems.

Over time, the colon or other parts of the gastrointestinal tract become inflamed, leading to increasingly worse symptoms. Justine fought symptoms of Crohn's disease for over fifteen years with pharmaceutical drugs like oxycodone, sulfasalazine, Pentasa, Remicade, Humira, Cimzia, Zofran, tramadol, prednisone, Flagyl, 6 MP, and Imuran, all of which failed to control her symptoms.

Now, she is proud that **cannabis juicing alone has put her disease into remission** and is doing everything she can to spread the word.

Justine Meader was diagnosed with Crohn's disease at age 13. After all pharmaceuticals failed her, she became a legal medicinal cannabis patient in Maine in 2011.

According to Justine, smoking cannabis helped alleviate nausea and pain to a small extent, but significant problems remained. Two years later, Justine learned about cannabis juicing from her boss at the dispensary where she worked. She and her husband studied the benefits of juicing, and decided it was the right course to take.

Justine acquired some cannabis leaves and bought a juicer. On June 13, 2013, she officially began juicing. **She began feeling better within seven days, and co-workers remarked on her increased energy.**

Previous blood work from May 24, 2013 indicated Justine's C-reactive protein level was 22, which is a sign of intense inflammation – a level of less than 8 is normal. **By July 12th, the CRP marker had dropped to 7.4.**

Before juicing, her symptoms included loss of appetite, diarrhea 10-12 times a day, and extreme fatigue. **Justine currently has none of those symptoms.** Furthermore, by November 4, 2014 multiple medical tests eventually showed **completely normal blood and a healthy colon.**

She concludes: "I am grateful to have found a way to alleviate my Crohn's symptoms naturally. The only side effect is my happiness."

Source: https://illegallyhealed.com/juicing-for-my-crohns-the-justine-meader-story

Case Study #88: Ulcerative Colitis No Match For Cannabis

"[Before Cannabis extracts]: Bloody, mucousy diarrhea daily and on Prednisone for five months straight; miserable, getting hives daily, mood swings, and very fatigued. Normal Ulcerative Colitis medications and Prednisone could not stop the flare. I was very concerned surgery to remove part of the colon may be the next step.

[After Cannabis extracts]: **I am off Prednisone, and no bloody, mucousy diarrhea anymore.** Cannabis Oil tincture labeled as Medium to High strength with coconut oil, the strains have varied depending on what's available, Sativas and hybrids mostly, a friend who is experienced with Oil processing and usages is making the oil for us.

In the beginning I started slowly working his way up to 15-25 drops daily, divided doses, taking the largest dose at bedtime. We also made capsules to use as suppositories, using them throughout the flare, now since the flare has subsided he is on a lower maintenance dosage of drops."

Source: www.cannabisoilsuccessstories.com/ulcerative-colitis.html

Case Study #89: Rare Bile Duct Condition Under Control Using Cannabis Oil

"My health was not good prior to using cannabis medicine. In 2011, I had a spinal fusion in my neck due to degenerative disc disease and was taking 90 mg of morphine a day. After the surgery I had no neck pain but after using morphine for 5 months, I was addicted to it. I was constantly having problems with my PSC and UC severe pain, cramping and nausea. Up to ten bowel movements a day with blood. I started having symptoms of EM but didn't know what it was until 2014.

Even though I'm on disability for my degenerative disc disease, I feel better now than before all my health issues started. **Cannabis helped me with the withdrawal symptoms after stopping morphine.** My liver tests are all normal now with no symptoms of PSC. **My Ulcerative Colitis has been under control with**

very few symptoms. My EM symptoms are less with cannabis.

I use a strain called AC/DC which is about 15% CBD and 0.5% THC, decarboxylated in the oven, ground up and put in gel capsules, 40mg three times a day. High THC oil 40mg once at night. A strain like Harlequin, vaporized 1:1 ratio THC to CBD, as needed for pain, nausea, cramping.

Dosing:
- CBD: 40mg gel capsule, orally, three times a day
- THC: 40mg gel capsule, orally, once at night
- Vaporized THC/CBD as needed
- CBD: 40mg gel capsule, orally, three times a day
- THC: 40mg gel capsule, orally, once at night
- Vaporized THC/CBD as needed

Other than marrying my wife, using cannabis has been the best decision I've ever made. It has given me my life back. I've lost 50 pounds, I exercise every day now and I feel great. I researched this medicine and its benefits extensively, there are thousands of scientific articles available on line. The disservice our federal Government has done to the American people by the prohibition of this wonderful medicine is unfathomable."

Source: www.cannabisoilsuccessstories.com/primary-sclerosing-cholangitis-treated-with-cannabis-oil.html

CHAPTER 21

Healing From Glaucoma

Glaucoma is a condition that many people associate with medicinal cannabis. In this chapter, I share four testimonials of people who have successfully treated Glaucoma with the help of cannabis.

Case Study #90: 58-Year-Old Woman Cures Her Cataracts and Glaucoma With Cannabis Extracts

A 58-year-old woman from Alabama cured her Glaucoma, as well as Cataracts and Arthritis, using Cannabis extracts. She states:

"I used reading glasses for the eye problems, and had arthritis pain throughout my body, including in my shoulder, and painful knots in my hands. I also had a staph infection. [I was taking] aspirin several times per day.

However, after taking Cannabis extract, **I no longer need reading glasses, no cataract surgery, no drops for glaucoma**, the knots in my hands are gone; all arthritis pain gone. I used oil to quit smoking cigarettes. The staph also healed. I got a hold of Sativa buds and made Cannabis Oil, using Everclear. I then mixed

189

some of the Cannabis Oil in a crock pot with coconut oil to make a topical.

I started with a small bead of Cannabis Oil on a teaspoon full of peanut butter. At first, I used it every 5-6 hours as needed for anxiety. I also used Cannabis Oil for the first three days when I quit smoking cigarettes cold-turkey, then used it three times daily. I used the Cannabis Oil-coconut oil mixture topically to clear up the staph infection.

On July 11, 2013 I went for an eye exam for reading glasses. The optometrist said, 'You know your health is not good right?' I knew I smoked way too much and was under weight, didn't eat right, so I just sat and listened to the doctor say this and that and then he noted the least of my problems were glaucoma and cataracts.

Three days later we made the Cannabis Oil and I used it to quit smoking cold-turkey after 40 years. After using the Cannabis Oil for two weeks I saw the referral doctor and she said no eye drops or surgery at that time. I no longer wear reading glasses either. **I have found Cannabis Oil heals most anything wrong with me,** as with my husband, who is 71 years of age."

Source: www.cannabisoilsuccessstories.com/cataracts---glaucoma.html

Case Study #91: Elvy Musikka Was Diagnosed With Glaucoma

"I was diagnosed with Glaucoma in 1975. Within a year, I already knew that there was nothing, **absolutely nothing that was on the market then worked for my glaucoma except for marijuana**... One of the benefits of using marijuana is that most of us drop all the other drugs that really do a number on our heads and make it difficult for us to stay healthy between our livers, kidneys and everything else about us. It takes other pills to take care of everything else. I don't have to deal with that. **I did discover marijuana and pretty soon I found that it was the only medicine I ever needed.**"

Source: www.leafly.com/news/health/cannabis-for-glaucoma-treatment

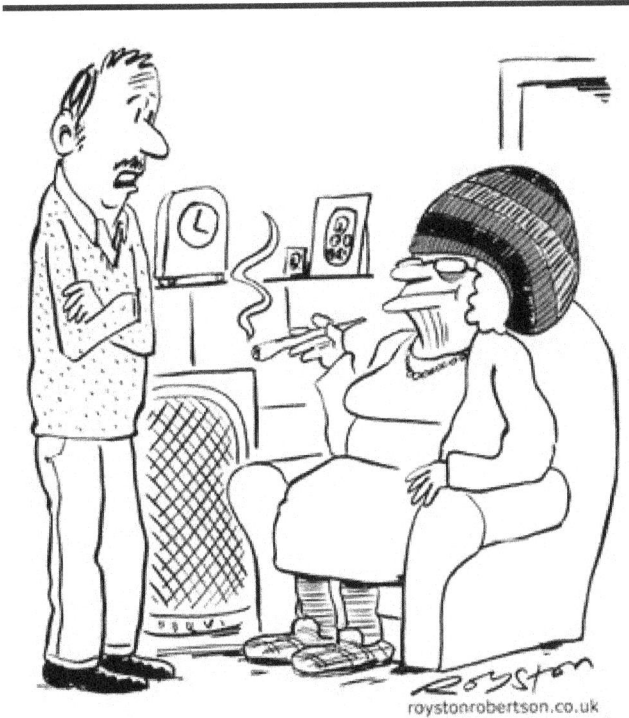

roystonrobertson.co.uk

"Mother, are you sure your marijuana use is purely medicinal?"

Case Study #92: Erin's Story (Glaucoma)

"After suffering a significant traumatic brain injury, Erin Delaney was diagnosed with Multiple Mechanism Glaucoma, a type of optic nerve damage with several difficult factors that make it hard to treat. With the help of her glaucoma specialist, she has explored every avenue to manage her condition's symptoms.

Like many people managing chronic conditions, Erin's medication list grew considerably over the years – from the prescriptions to treat her glaucoma to the medications intended to mitigate some of the side effects of her glaucoma meds, and so on. At one point, Erin thought to herself, "I'm too young to be on so many pills."

The conventional treatments weren't as effective as Erin's care team had hoped, and after further study the team concluded that the same brain injury that provoked the condition was overriding the treatments. A significant pressure attack brought Erin to her glaucoma specialist for a conversation about a new treatment plan.

During a pressure attack, pressure on the optic nerve increases rapidly and dramatically, often causing headaches and nausea. Pressure attacks may be triggered by small changes in the weather or a change in the patient's activity level. Some glaucoma patients can tell if a pressure attack is about to happen and take medications to forestall the side effects. Yet, in addition to the pain and nausea, there is fear: **"one attack is all it takes to completely cut off circulation to the optic nerve,"
Erin explained. The result would be blindness.**

Once cleared by the state, Erin made an appointment at LeafLine Labs. "If you had told me two years ago that I would be on medical marijuana, I would have laughed you out of the room," Erin said. "Like many, I thought it was just a bunch of 'potheads' looking for a legal loophole." Her sentiment has since changed.

Walking through the doors for the first time, Erin remembers, "the facility itself felt like a dignified, serious clinical setting. I learned that my phenomenal pharmacist used to work with the neurologist who treated my aneurysm. His knowledge of the protocols in place and the context let me know he was 'on it,' which was a huge relief."

Erin also toured the production facilities where the cannabis plants are grown, oils extracted, and medicine crafted. Learning of the credentials and backgrounds of the lab team, Erin remarked, "I was both blown away and not at all surprised to see all of the protocols and care that go into the extraction process. They are committed to producing a product of consistently high quality."

After considering her options, Erin decided to try the Heather vaporizer oil cartridges; a product with a 1:1 ratio of THC to CBD. "I wanted to start light, a decision my pharmacist respected," said Erin. "Initially I was concerned about mood alterations and possible side effects; I've got a 7-year-old to keep up with!"

Within a few minutes of taking Heather, Erin can feel the pressure easing. She has even measured a 7-point drop in her optic nerve pressure at her doctor's office. Erin has been able to keep her optic pressure readings low enough on Heather to qualify for additional surgical procedures to treat her glaucoma.

Erin notes that Heather is not a cure nor a replacement – but rather it is a key component in her integrated care plan that **has helped her reduce the number of her prescribed medications by 50 percent.** "For treating the secondary symptoms of my pressure attacks, I now vape for nearly instant relief. Before I would have taken pills that would take time to go into effect and still leave me with stomach aches and ulcers. Medications are expensive already but add in the side effects and over time you question their true value to your quality of life."

Source: https://leaflinelabs.com/patient-firsts/2017/6/20/medical-cannabis-glaucoma-erins-story

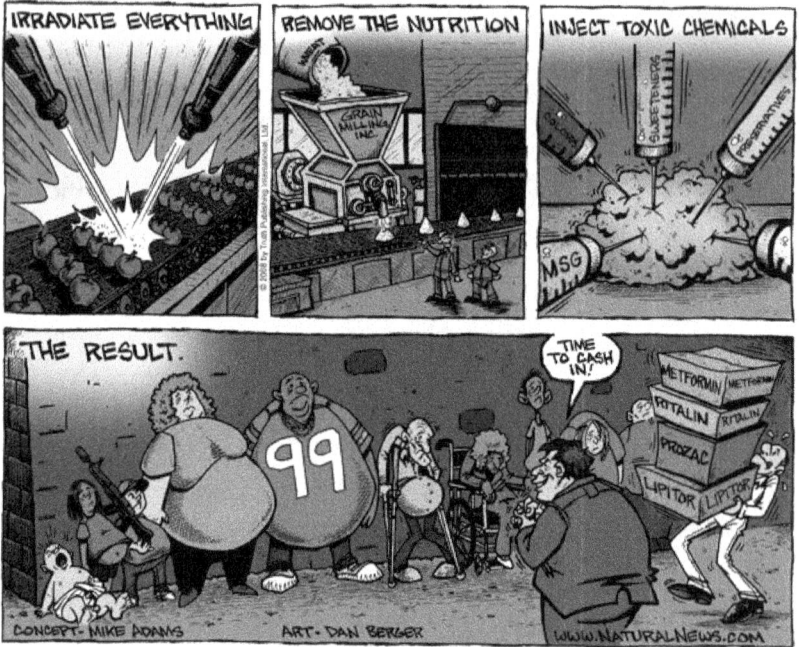

Thanks to Mike Adams and *www.NaturalNews.com* for the cartoon above

CHAPTER 22

Amyotrophic Lateral Sclerosis (ALS) and Cannabis

In this chapter, I share the stories of two incredible individuals who used cannabis extracts to help treat ALS. You'll learn about their journey back to health as well as their thoughts and experiences in using this natural remedy.

Case Study #93: Bob Striders Conquers ALS By Taking His Healing In His Own Hands

"Amyotrophic lateral sclerosis (ALS) is one of the most degenerative motor neuron diseases in existence. Most people with ALS die within three to five years after symptom onset, and the disease often progresses very rapidly. Bob Strider wants others to know **this prognosis is not written in stone**, and cannabis can be a truly effective option for many ALS patients.

Bob has had an especially storied life. He graduated from Harvard University, and from 1965 to 1969 acted as a voice intercept operator for the United States Army, working out of Germany to monitor Russian communications. In 1991, Bob moved to the capital of the Czech Republic, Prague, where he essentially remained for two decades. The environment was very supportive of Bob's passion for biking, and he often put in 400 kilometres a week.

In 1998, Bob began experiencing the first symptoms of ALS. These symptoms included a loss of function in his right arm and problems swallowing.

By 2012, his overall health had gotten really bad, and **Bob knew he had to try something better**. He had been smoking large amounts of cannabis for years, which he believed was responsible for the slow progression of the disease. However, Bob felt cannabis oil would work even better.

Bob literally took his healing into his own hands. In 2012, he set up two grow rooms and a lab in order to produce cannabis oil. This was especially difficult given Bob's limited mobility, but hope fuelled his physical labour and he had a lot of help from friends.

Once he had produced cannabis oil, Bob began with a quarter gram per day. Within the next week he quickly escalated his daily intake to half a gram, then a full gram.

Due to his lifelong use of psychoactive cannabis, Bob was able to accelerate his dosing regimen faster than most patients. He continued at a gram a day for about 60 days before beginning to use a lower dose due to supply concerns.

Within 10 days, Bob had his right arm back, and could even throw a football. His overall condition improved tremendously. **He stopped using all pharmaceuticals, including the codeine and aspirin** he needed for pain. Unlike pills, the oil had a number of remarkable side effects. The high blood pressure Bob had struggled with for years completely dropped, to the point where he had to control his oil intake to make sure it did not get too low.

Indeed, CB1 activation is linked with hypotensive effects. **Nummular eczema, asthma, and a herpes infection also all disappeared**. Scientific studies indicate the potential of cannabinoids to benefit these conditions through bronco-dilatory, anti-inflammatory, and anti-viral capabilities. Also, a January 2015 review implicated cannabinoids in the potential treatment of many neuroinflammatory disorders, including ALS.

In September 2014, Bob returned to Massachusetts, partially because he wanted to share what he had learned about treating ALS with cannabis. While Bob still has problems with swallowing and some other symptoms, he says **continued treatment almost makes him feel like he is getting younger**. He believes that if he can increase his dose of decarboxylated and raw, acidic cannabinoids, he can more completely reverse the disease.

One reason Bob is excited about the potential of raw cannabinoids, and cannabis extracts as a whole, is due to the experience of one of his friends in Prague. **The friend had been diagnosed with Stage IV melanoma that had spread to his liver and brain**.

He began simmering the bottom leaves of cannabis in milk at a low heat all day, creating an infusion. For years he continuously drank the milk and rubbed it on the surface-level lesions. **Six years later he is cancer free**, and the only treatment he used was that milk preparation.

The ability of an ALS patient to survive decades beyond the expected lifespan is also not unique. A Florida patient named Cathy Jordan is almost **30 years into her ALS diagnosis**, a feat she attributes to cannabis.

It is critical that patients are not restricted in how much cannabis they can access. For people with seriously advanced illnesses, they often need several ounces of raw cannabis a month to ingest the necessary quantities of oil and raw juice. When patients have access to the right medicines at the right quantities, truly miraculous things can happen."

Source:https://turnthingsupsidedown.wordpress.com/2016/09/10/illegally-healed-from-als

Case Study #94: Cathy Jordan Defies the Odds

Cathy Jordan, who was diagnosed with ALS in 1986 and given less than five years to live. In the winter of 1989, Jordan spent the holiday in Florida, preparing for the end of her life, when she made a crucial discovery. While walking on the beach one night, **she smoked a joint of Myakka Gold and felt her symptoms cease,** essentially experiencing the neuroprotective effects of cannabis before they'd been proven.

Jordan never set out to be a cannabis activist, preferring instead to quietly continue treating her disease. She tried to tell her neurologist in 1989 that cannabis had helped her, and he tried to convince her husband to have her committed to a mental facility.

In 1994, **Jordan met a new doctor who was astonished by her progress.** When he asked what she'd been doing to stay alive, she informed him, and he advised her, "Smoke all the cannabis you can and never tell a soul, because they will never believe you."

Source: www.leafly.com/news/science-tech/the-medical-minute-how-does-cannabis-impact-the-progression-of-al

CHAPTER 23

Anxiety, Depression, PTSD, and Chronic Fatigue

Anxiety disorders, depression, and chronic fatigue can be debilitating. Although the solution put forward by the Medical Establishment often involves pharmaceutical drugs, this chapter presents testimonials from numerous people who successfully treated their symptoms using little more than cannabis extracts.

Case Study #95: 70-Year-Old Carol Francey Campaigns for Cannabis Legislation

"Vancouver resident Carol Francey attributes cannabis use of more than five decades to her excellent health today. According to Francey, she smoked cannabis **to alleviate various conditions such as arthritis, sciatica, and insomnia**. Francey added that her previous medications used to affect her balance and slurred her speech. However, the use of various forms of cannabis proved helpful in relieving her conditions without the unwanted side effects from her medications.

"**I threw away all my pills**. They had slurred my speech and affected my balance. Now [I have] a little concentrated oil which relaxes, soothes, repairs, and prevents illnesses. A hot coffee with a toasty cannabis tincture works well for arthritis, pain, and sleep. [I'll inhale] a dab for sciatica and I'm after that I can walk...**We need to help older people have a better quality of life.** Cannabis helps you to overcome anxiety about day-to-day life and stop sweating the small stuff," Francey said in a *Daily Mail* article.

Francey first started using cannabis at the age of 17 but did not disclose it publicly for fears of social stigma, and how the activity would affect her reputation as a former drugs and alcohol counsellor. The grandmother campaigned for cannabis legislation in the country with the group 'Grannies for Grass International' and is encouraging other cannabis users to come out in the open.

A vast number of studies have demonstrated the many beneficial effects of cannabis use. For instance, a comprehensive meta-analysis published in the journal *Clinical Psychology Review* revealed that **taking medical cannabis is beneficial for the treatment of post-traumatic stress disorder (PTSD), social anxiety, and depression**.

A team of researchers examined 31 studies as part of the review and found that the cannabidiol compound in cannabis contained potent antidepressant and anti-anxiety effects. Likewise, the compound helped inhibit continuous retrieval of a traumatic event in patients with PTSD. The compound was also known to relieve stress and anxiety in PTSD patients. Moreover, cannabidiol was found to outperform opiates in keeping alcohol- and opioid-dependent patients off their addictions.

"We are really excited about the potential substitution effect. If people use cannabis as a replacement for opioid medications, or to get off of opioids or cut back, we could see some pretty dramatic public health benefits. The level of opioid overdoses is so high right now. I think people will derive more benefits if they can speak more openly with providers about whether they are using cannabis and why," lead researcher Zach Walsh said."

Source: www.newstarget.com/2018-01-03-cannabis-more-effective-than-prescriptions-seventy-year-old-grandmother-threw-out-all-her-pills-says-smoking-cannabis-manages-her-ailments.html

Case Study #96: Joseph's Pain, Night Terrors, Panic Attacks, Stomach Problems, and Schizophrenia Symptoms Drop Dramatically Thanks To Cannabis Use

"Joseph has dealt with a lot in his relatively short life. From birth, he was diagnosed with neurofibromatosis type I (NF-1), a genetic disorder that can cause tumours in the nervous system along with other symptoms like seizures.

Fighting this disease has led to potentially related problems later in life, including schizophrenia, post-traumatic stress disorder, and stomach problems. While pharmaceuticals have been somewhat effective, their side effects have left a lot to be desired.

Joseph is currently 20 years old, and it was not until he went to college that he tried cannabis. His roommate introduced him to the plant, and **Joseph instantly realized how therapeutically effective it was**. Smoking cannabis benefits virtually all of his symptoms. **Night terrors and panic attacks have substantially reduced, as have anxiety symptoms. Pain measures and other assorted symptoms have also dropped dramatically.**

In addition to traditional metrics, Joseph's general **quality of life has remarkably improved.** When not using cannabis, he is very anti-social and has trouble talking with people. This problem is almost non-existent with cannabis, which also reduces his general stress levels.

Another interesting feature of using cannabis is how it benefits Joseph's schizophrenia. **He says cannabis makes it like the schizophrenia is not there, and he will not see the "triggers" that activate symptoms.** Compared to pharmaceuticals, no matter what the symptom is, Joseph says cannabis "just works better".

"Cannabis is more effective and also lacks the side effects of chemical medications." Says Joseph.

Neural activity is arguably linked to all of Joseph's symptoms. Therefore, it is no surprise that cannabis has proven so beneficial. Cannabinoids are known to benefit the nervous system through neuroprotective, antioxidant and pro-neurogenesis properties.

Furthermore, components of cannabis like cannabidiol (CBD) **have been proven in double-blind, randomized clinical trials to benefit schizophrenia.** Whole-plant cannabis has been linked to reduced neuropathic pain as well.

It is hopeful that as the legal environment further changes, Joseph will have access to higher-quality cannabis extracts that will deliver even better results than the phenomenal improvements he has already experienced."

Source: https://illegallyhealed.com/finding-inner-peace

Case Study #97: Chad Lozano Moves On From PTSD, Anxiety, Paranoia and Anger Thanks to Cannabis

"Chad Lozano is an Iraq war veteran who has found cannabis to be more effective than traditional medicines, and he wants to do everything in his power to help other struggling veterans.

Chad was almost literally bred to be in the military, as he was born at Holloman Air Force Base. Although he was initially planning to join the Air Force, his sister convinced him to go into the Army instead. He joined at age 21 in 2008, graduating basic training in May and being deployed to Iraq in March 2009 as Army Intel.

Within three hours of getting to Iraq his unit was mortared, which instantly impressed Chad with the reality that he was in a war zone. He did a nine-month tour and returned to Hawaii in November 2009, where he remained with the Army until leaving in July 2011.

Within this time, Chad endured trauma from numerous sources. In Iraq, he lost friends and saw many of the terrible things associated with war. At home, he lost two uncles. After returning home, he also lost his sister to prescription pills in 2010, which she had been using as a result of her earlier Army experience.

Until he got home, Chad did not realize the extent to which all his experiences had affected him. He was angry, paranoid, and had trouble sleeping. He eventually realized he needed help but did not want to turn to pills because of what happened to his sister.

He had heard positive things about medicinal cannabis, so he conducted research and learned the plant was actually prescribed for PTSD in New Mexico, where his family lived. In 2013 he joined the New Mexico medicinal cannabis program.

Once Chad began using cannabis, he quickly saw how beneficial it was. It helps him sleep and has almost eliminated his anxiety, paranoia, and anger. Overall, cannabis contributes to a state of calmness. Thanks to the medicine, Chad is in an excellent state of health and needs no pharmaceuticals to control what otherwise might have been a severe case of PTSD.

It's not only thousands of Vets that attest to the efficacy of cannabis. According to a study published in the journal *Neuropsychopharmacology*, research suggest that the connectivity within the brain's fear circuit changes following trauma, and the administration of cannabinoids prevents this change from happening."

Source: https://illegallyhealed.com/the-rise-of-vets-using-cannabis-for-ptsd

Case Study #98: Hollywood Actresses Jennifer Aniston and Olivia Wilde Use CBD Oil to Relieve Pain, Stress and Anxiety

"The National Institute on Drug Abuse determined after several studies that CBD oil reduces stress in animals, and that they exhibited fewer behavioural signs of anxiety after being treated with the oil.

And, in 2011, the Journal of Psychopharmacology published a study which found that 400 milligrams of CBD effectively **reduced symptoms of anxiety in patients with Seasonal Affective Disorder (SAD).**

Countless other studies have reached the same conclusion: When it comes to anxiety, CBD oil works.

The Anxiety Centre reports that around 18.1 percent of all American adults are diagnosed with some form of anxiety, though experts believe that the true figure is closer to 30 percent, since many people do not seek help for the condition. A study commissioned by the Anxiety and Depression Association of America (ADAA) found that anxiety disorders cost the country over $42 billion each year – a third of all the costs associated with mental health in the U.S.

Big Pharma's go-to drugs for anxiety are selective serotonin reuptake inhibitors (SSRIs) like Zoloft and Prozac. However, these dangerous drugs cause multiple side effects, and an increasing number of people – including celebrities – are turning to a natural, safe alternative to cope with their anxiety called cannabidiol (CBD) oil.

CBD is an oil that is sourced from the hemp plant – a variety of the Cannabis Sativa plant that is grown specifically for industrial uses in the production of paper, clothing, biodegradable plastics, etc. Unlike the cannabinoid tetrahydrocannabinol (THC) found in marijuana, CBD does not have any psychoactive properties and does not produce a high. It is both legal and safe.

The exact way CBD affects CB1 is not fully understood. However, it's thought that it alters serotonin signals. Serotonin is one of your body's chemicals and plays a role in your mental health. Low serotonin levels are common in depression. Not having enough serotonin can also cause anxiety in some people.

Dr. Sarah Brewer, a GP and the medical director of the company Healthspan, noted that CBD oil has noticeably beneficial psychological effects and reduces anxiety while promoting relaxation and a good night's sleep.

Healthista reported recently that countless celebrities, including Jennifer Aniston, sing the praises of CBD oil when it comes to treating stress, pain and anxiety. **"CBD helps with pain, stress and anxiety," Aniston told US Weekly.**

And actress Olivia Wilde told the New York Times that she uses a body lotion infused with CBD oil and finds that it helps her to relax. She believes it also helps her to avoid using chemical painkillers when her work causes her back and neck pain."

Source: www.naturalnews.com/2018-05-23-cbd-oil-a-miracle-oil-that-helps-with-anxiety-with-no-high.html

Case Study #99: Anxiety and Muscle Spasms Eased With Cannabis Extracts

"I was waking up almost every night with severe panic attacks worrying about everything from work, my kids, money, getting up to double-check that the doors and windows were all locked, etc. Heart racing, parts of body feeling numb, and not being able to get back to sleep for a couple hours. I was also experiencing muscle spasms in my feet and calves.

After taking Cannabis extracts, I'm sleeping great and having very few anxiety episodes. Muscle cramps are gone.

I take coconut oil infused with Full Extract Cannabis Oil, high in THC, random strains of Cannabis flowers and various edibles. Ten drops of tincture 2-3 times per day, with one of the doses right before bed; Two to three hits from a pipe, twice per day, with one session about an hour before bed; I eat edibles only on vacation because they are easier to conceal than flower and a pipe.

Cannabis has helped me to feel normal again. I just feel better with cannabis in my system! I highly (pun intended) recommend it to anyone experiencing these symptoms."

Source: www.cannabisoilsuccessstories.com/anxiety---muscle-spasms.html

Case Study #100: AIDS and Major Depression Under Control Without Pharmaceuticals

"Since early adolescence I experienced extreme depression and was diagnosed with Major Depressive Disorder. I have been on scores of pharmaceutical anti-depressants to treat my depression and have attempted suicide countless times.

In September of 2011 I was diagnosed with HIV/AIDS and cryptococcal meningitis. When I opened my mouth, it looked like I was The Crypt Keeper as I was full of thrush and the lining of my brain was being taken over by yeast. My T-cell count was 7.

Although smoking cannabis daily to treat depression helped my HIV go undetected for up to ten years and progress to AIDS **I credit both cannabis oil and ingestion of raw cannabis for allowing me to maintain a degree of health I'd be unable to maintain otherwise.**

It took only nine months from my diagnosis using pharmaceutical antiretroviral therapy and any and all forms of cannabis available to me to get to an undetectable viral load, although that has fluctuated through my last five years living with AIDS as I tried experimental treatments.

I'm happy to be free of pharmaceutical antidepressants and use cannabis and exercise as my only antidepressants now. I've found that the pharmaceutical antidepressants numbed me emotionally, dulled my life experience, and caused me to experience a medical emergency called brain shivers if and when I ran out of those medications. Using cannabis also allows me to maintain adherence to my pharmaceutical antiretroviral regimen by helping manage side effects from those medications like nausea, headache, etc!

I quit my job as a unit secretary on an oncology unit at a reputable hospital during the summer of 2013 and I've now been making cannabis oil for at least three years. I extract from primarily high THC cannabis material using 190 proof grain alcohol and a distiller. I blend with coconut or olive oil in varying dosage concentrations and put into capsules and glass bottles for sublingual drops. I use low and medium dose capsules during the day and take high dose capsules at night to sleep and I smoke dried flower through the day. Sometimes I also use an infused topical oil, and I eat at least a few raw Cannabis leaves daily or in a Budwig smoothie.

For many years to treat depression I smoked approximately 1/2 an ounce of dried Cannabis per month. Now I take approximately 2-4 grams of Cannabis Oil (in the form of capsules and sublingual drops) and smoke approximately 3/4 to one ounce of dried flower per month. Monthly intake of raw Cannabis leaves would be approximately an ounce.

I have good quality of life and am thankful for every day. Cannabis is helping save/extend my life."

Source:
www.cannabisoilsuccessstories.com/aids-and-major-depression.html

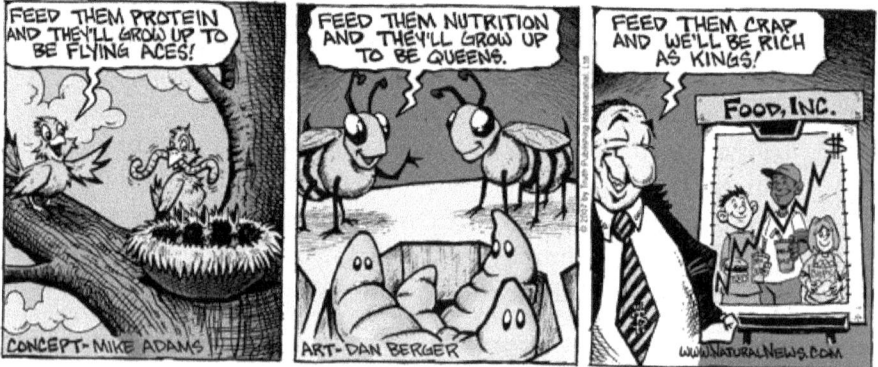

Thanks to Mike Adams and *www.NaturalNews.com* for the cartoon above.

Case Study #101: Fifteen-Year-Old Tom Bethell's Remarkable Turnaround From Chronic Fatigue

"A British teenager beset by chronic fatigue syndrome has made a remarkable recovery with the help of cannabis oil. Fifteen-year-old Tom Bethell had not been to school in almost eight years due to the illness and the severe depression that it caused.

Weak and bed-ridden, the young man stopped growing and his eye muscles didn't function properly, causing blurred vision. Nothing seemed to help, and he told his mother that he no longer wished to live.

According to his mother, he had no energy and appeared to be in a complete "brain fog." Falling as many as 20 or 30 times per day, he was unable to breathe correctly. After failed medications including antidepressants, his desperate mother turned to cannabis oil after her own mother found relief from Crohn's disease with it.

Once the teenager started taking the oil, his turn-around was almost immediately apparent. He grew a remarkable 11 inches in just nine months, and his hair, which had long stopped growing, began to grow once again. He finally went through puberty, growing leg and body hair. His feet grew two shoe sizes in two months.

His memory has improved, and he's gone from being unable to carry a conversation to preparing for high school exams. **The CBD has given him a chance to be himself and has eliminated his reactive depression.**

Now very much a happy and typical 15-year-old, his mother said: "Never in my wildest dreams did I expect to see him like this."

Source: www.naturalnews.com/2018-01-04-cannabis-oil-for-chronic-fatigue-a-teenager-says-it-cured-his-debilitating-illness.html

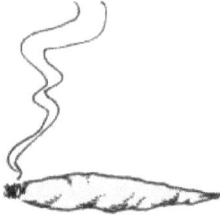

MEDICAL MARIJUANA

THIS SIMPLE DRIED HERB IS ILLEGAL

HOWEVER, IF A MULTINATIONAL DRUG COMPANY GRINDS UP THAT HERB, EXTRACTS THE CANNABIS SATIVA AND CREATES SYNTHETIC DELTA-9-TETRAHYDROCANNABI-NOL, COMBINES IT WITH GELATIN, GLYCERIN, IRON OXIDE RED, IRON OXIDE YELLOW, TITANIUM DIOXIDE, MARKETS IT TO DOCTORS AND HOSPITALS UNDER THE NAME MARINOL AND IN THE PROCESS MAKES A BUNCH OF WEALTHY WALL STREET INVESTORS EVEN RICHER, THEN IT'S LEGAL.

© HARTFORD COURANT.

CHAPTER 24

Alzheimer's and Parkinson's Disease

The following stories are from people suffering with Parkinson's and Alzheimer's disease who have found cannabis extracts extremely beneficial and want to share their experiences with the world.

The evidence is strong that regular, moderate use of cannabis helps to delay the onset and progression of neurodegenerative conditions, as the following case studies can attest to.

Case Study #102: Sheriff's Deputy Quits to Treat Parkinson's with Cannabis

"Richard Secklin has led a remarkably storied life. Growing up in Milwaukee, Wisconsin, he started his career as a professional bodybuilder after returning from a four-year enlistment in the U.S. Navy. Richard eventually moved to New Mexico and opened his own gym, which he successfully managed for several years.

Richard started working in law enforcement at a correctional facility. Eventually, he moved to Texas to continue his career as a Sheriff's Deputy. He went back to school and got a degree in organizational management, which helped him rise to the rank of Sergeant and become an instructor.

At age 50 in 2003, while graduating from college, Richard was diagnosed with Parkinson's disease. He began taking the standard medications for the disease, which caused some unpleasant side effects. Richard's ex-wife knew about the benefits of cannabis for Parkinson's and brought him a joint in 2005. He found smoking cannabis tremendously helped the Parkinson's symptoms.

For several months Richard hid his use of cannabis and kept working, but eventually realized he needed to focus on his own healing. Therefore, he left his job in law enforcement and moved back to Wisconsin.

Leaving Texas worked out well for Richard. He has been able to use higher amounts of cannabis, as his access had been severely limited. His method of ingestion is vaporization at night. One time, he tried an industrial hemp-derived cannabidiol (CBD) oil which he says reduced his right knee pain and improved his sleep. Other than that, all the cannabis Richard has used has been predominantly rich in tetrahydrocannabinol (THC).

Richard believes his cannabis use has significantly slowed down the progression of his disease. Most other Parkinson's patients he knows have to go into nursing homes 4 or 5 years after initial diagnosis. **Richard is still independent 11 years after diagnosis.**

The primary traditional medicine he uses is Levadopa, but he does not need antidepressants or pain medication. Cannabis has also potentially replaced sleeping pills, as when Richard uses the medicine he can sleep 6-7 hours through the night. On the whole, Richard says cannabis has been 'immensely helpful'.

THC has been shown to exert exceptional neuroprotective effects. One study indicated it protected against three different Parkinson's disease-relevant toxins. Interestingly, CBD was unable to elicit the same neuroprotection as THC. However, a double-blind trial conducted in 2014 pointed to the potential of CBD to improve quality of life in Parkinson's patients. According to researchers, the lesser-known cannabinoid tetrahydrocannabivarin (THCV) may also help delay disease progression.

Richard has an active blog and has written two books about his journey with cannabis. Including, 'Marijuana for Parkinson's Disease' and 'Parkinson's Disease: Looking Down the Barrel'."

Source: https://illegallyhealed.com/sheriffs-deputy-quits-to-treat-parkinsons-with-cannabis/

Case Study #103: Marie Van Tonder Gets Tremors Under Control with Cannabis

"I cannot imagine what my life would have been without Cannabis oil treatment. I have been on chronic medicine from 1995 for Thyroid and high blood pressure. About 7 years ago I was diagnosed with a familial tremor and told there was nothing they could do for me. I was then diagnosed with Parkinson's... and that was when I started using Cannabis oil.

I am off all medicines now for 5 months without any problems!

The lady who does my nails every six weeks, told me she can't believe the improvement of the tremor especially in both my thumbs which were really bad. I can now use a fork and knife instead of a spoon when eating. The left hand still sometimes is a bit awkward when I am in a hurry or anxious or when a lot of people are present. But overall my condition is so much better.

I am so grateful for all your help… I don't have words to express my gratitude. Thanks to the Cannabis Oil Research team! May you all be blessed in helping others like me!"

Source: www.cannabisoilresearch.com/testimonials/parkinsons-disease

Case Study #104: Larry Smith's Severe Dyskinesia, Loss of Voice, and Tremors Are Calmed Within Minutes

"Former police officer Larry Smith began seeing the effects of the Parkinson's disease 20 years ago and his health has been declining ever since. After two decades of attempting a variety of treatments and seeing no substantial results, he turned to medical marijuana as a last resort.

In the first video, he speaks with a doctor who is able to provide a medical marijuana card and allow Larry to purchase the treatment. When the doctor asks Larry how he's been feeling lately, Larry responds by saying, "My symptoms are a great deal more obvious than ever before, and the pain is a little sharper."

Larry suffers greatly from dyskinesia, which is a category of movement by involuntary muscle movements, and has trouble walking and speaking. His wife said that he has so much trouble with walking that he now takes 20 pills every day. The medication he takes costs upwards of $3,000, but when he arrives at a medical marijuana dispensary, he pays only $40 for his first dosage of marijuana buds.

"With a few drops of cannabis oil under his tongue, Larry's severe dyskinesia (uncontrolled movements), loss of voice and tremors are calmed within minutes! We didn't even edit the footage because the results were so startling."

Immediately after administering the treatment, he stands up with no problem and says, "A person like me could really use marijuana and it makes me pretty angry that I can't get it in my home state."

His home state of South Dakota does not allow for the use of medical marijuana, which is why Larry and his wife travelled to San Diego to receive the treatment.

The former cop has since decided to train and complete a 300-mile bike ride across South Dakota, a feat that the filmmakers, who are filming Ride With Larry, plan to capture."

Source: http://www.trueactivist.com/watch-former-cop-shocked-after-treating-parkinsons-symptoms-with-cannabis

DeATHS FROM ALCoHoL

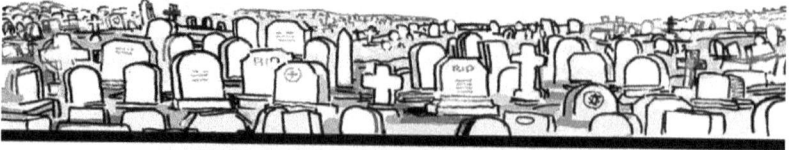

DeATHS FROM CiGAReTTes

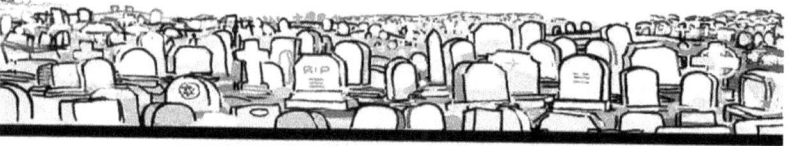

DeATHS FROM MARiJuANA

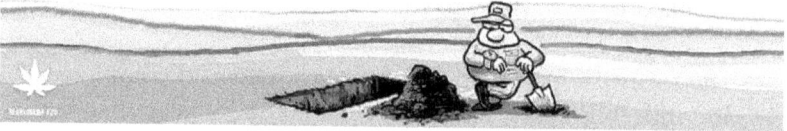

Case Study #105: Alzheimer's Sufferer
Finding New Life with Cannabis Oil

"My 96-year-old patient was basically catatonic. Staring at her hands or down at the floor. Hasn't spoken in over five years, makes no eye contact or attempt to communicate. Only noise made is during restless sleep throughout the night. Has to have everything done for her.

The patient is in good health other than Alzheimer's, only medications are as needed when a problem arises.

First night on [Cannabis] oil, sleep was noticeably more peaceful and has been since. Each day that passes she is also noticeably more alert. Eyes stay wide open and she looks around the room and at you when you speak to her or touch her, and she makes eye contact regularly now. Still can't speak sentences but is trying to communicate. Will put four or five random words toge-ther at a time or make a happy excited run of what

216

sounds like a shrill hum and then followed with the word 'Yeah' and a smile. **She hasn't done these things in five years!** At her age and considering how advanced the Alzheimer's was when she started, the goal was to at least give her quality. Maybe have her be able to say 'yes' or 'no' or give some indication of her comfort level. We're not there yet but it's only been a little over a month, so the outlook is promising.

[She is given] one grain of rice sized dose once daily; after dinner with dessert.

This is not my story but one I'm proud to say I'm responsible for because I educated her caregiver on Cannabis oil. The oil improved the quality of my own life so much I do my best to spread the word everywhere I go. This particular patient has a personal, live-in caregiver who made the choice to try it for her and we're both enjoying watching her gradually regain her lucidity a little more each day!"

Source: www.cannabisoilsuccessstories.com/alzheimer-s-sufferer-finds-hope-in-cannabis.html

Case Study #106: 79-Year-Old Alzheimer's Sufferer Taken Off Valium

"My wife, at age 79, had all the symptoms of Alzheimer's with sleep disturbance, depression, impaired judgement, anxiety, frustration, behavioural changes, loss of appetite, migraines and nausea.

My wife now has a solid nine hours sleep per night with two toilet breaks and has two one-hour naps during the day. She now eats everything given her with snacks in between, has only slight headaches and less nausea. Her depression, anxiety and frustration has now become her old self of a sense of humour and smiles again. I'm pleased and happy with that because everything else I can live with.

Because of the success of the Cannabis Oil, I have successfully weaned my wife off the Valium."

Source:www.cannabisoilsuccessstories.com/alzheimer-s-in-australia.html

Case Study #107: Alzheimer's Under Control For 92 Year-Old California Woman

"I'm writing this for my mother. At about age 85, she was diagnosed with dementia and later Alzheimer's. At close to 90, she had a stroke leaving her in a wheelchair and unable to speak. The Alzheimer's medications she got left her unresponsive. She looked stunned, unable to speak and teary-eyed. The stroke also left her arms and legs permanently bent.

Our Cannabis Oil journey started out as an accident. I use Cannabis Oil for my arthritic fingers. We would occasionally use it on my mother's arms which have started to shrivel up due to the stroke. **We notice that after a few minutes of rubbing in the Cannabis Oil, her stiff arms would get softer.** From then on, we started giving her Cannabis Oil rubs followed by arm stretching daily.

After researching some more, we decided to give her Cannabis Oil orally, in lieu of the medications. We slowly weened her off the medications until all she was getting was Cannabis Oil. **Today at age 92, she has started to speak again,** although mumbling. From time to time, her words would be accurately clear and in the correct context. She smiles and laughs a lot now and has good eye contact. Her arms before were locked close to her chest. Now we can move it past the 90-degree angle without the previous pain she encountered.

To date, her daily regiment is taking two Cannabis chocolate candies in the morning with a Cannabis Oil massage, two teaspoons of a slightly stronger Cannabis Oil before bed time to giver the deep sleep she needs. When she gets agitated mid-day, we give her one or two chocolate candies as needed.

We make our own cannabis oil. We use a strain called Durga Mata 2 which has about 7% CBD / 7% THC. Our formula for the base oil is basically steeping 10 grams of cannabis flowers for every cup of coconut oil for about 4 to 8 hours in very slow heat (crackpot). From this base oil, we add chocolate bars and then pour it into a mold.

Ten grams (10,000mg) of Cannabis Oil with 7% THC and 7% CBD will yield 700 milligrams of CBD and 700 milligrams of THC. When mixed into a cup of coconut oil (48 teaspoons per cup), each teaspoon will have 14.6 milligrams of THC and 14.6 milligrams of CBD (700 milligrams divide by 48 teaspoons). I hope my math is correct.

At night, we give my mother about a teaspoon of the coconut oil mix. In the morning, we give her a candy bar the size of a teaspoon. The chocolate bars just giver some variety. We've also observed that a stronger heat when cooking the oil gives more of a sedative effect. For her morning candy, we cook it in a double boiler where temp of the oil hovers about 200 deg F. For her evening oil, we use a direct heat in low setting where the oil temp is about 240 deg F. The night time oil makes her sleepy. I try the oil on myself before giving it to her.

When we started out, there was a lot of push back even from family members. We had one family member who even tried to kill her plants. We got her a license at age 90 just to make sure nobody can say we were putting her in harm's way. Now with her starting to mumble and interact again, the push back has disappeared. **There is a lot of ignorance when it comes to this helpful plant.** I think the plant has very high anti-inflammatory and high antioxidant properties. Most of the ailments are inflammation and oxidation occurring in the body. Think of the plant as herbal medicine that has been used for thousands of years before it was persecuted by governments bribed by big corporations."

Source: www.cannabisoilsuccessstories.com/alzheimer-s--92-yo-female.html

FINAL THOUGHTS

While government regulations and the scientific community play catch-up to the overwhelming evidence available today about the extraordinary healing propertics of the cannabis plant, we should do everything in our power to disseminate the inspiring stories contained in this book as far and as wide as possible.

Share them with your friends, your loved ones, and your community. Share them on social media. Share this book with your doctor or health-care practitioner. Get the word out there. A revolution in the healthcare industry is afoot.

Remember, when you embark on your journey back to health, that while cannabis in itself may help you tremendously along the way, maintaining healthy habits such as exercising daily and getting sound sleep, detoxifying your system, consuming organic food and using the best available supplements, also go a long way, as does maintaining a positive mental attitude. Often, discovering the mental and emotional root cause of a disease is the first step in truly eliminating that health problem from our lives permanently (check out the work of British researcher Richard Moat on this topic).

Lastly, please do share with me in due course your story of getting back to health – your very own "Cannabis Miracle."

Feel free to get in touch via email at info@prosperitypower.com.

I look forward to hearing from you soon!

To Your Happiness & Success,

Mark Anastasi

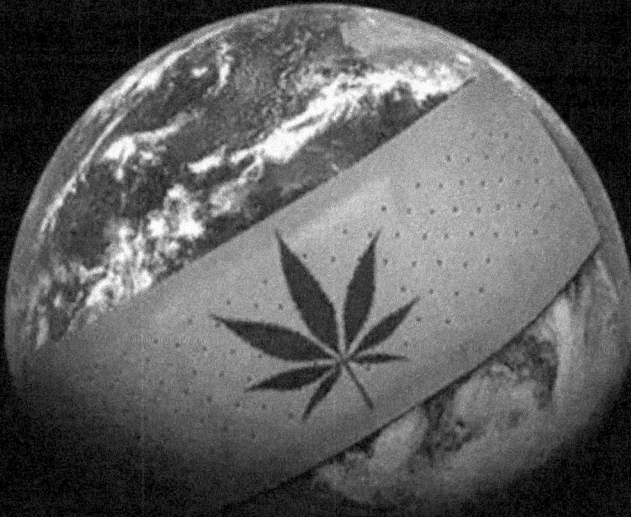

"I don't know if hemp's gonna save the world, but I'll tell you this ...

...it's the only thing that can."
– Jack Herer.

www.ingramcontent.com/pod-product-compliance
Lightning Source LLC
Chambersburg PA
CBHW071019280326

41935CB00011B/1423